Health Promotion Practice

Health Promotion Practice

Power and Empowerment

Glenn Laverack

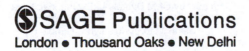

SAGE Publications

London • Thousand Oaks • New Delhi

ISBN 0-7619-4179-7 (hbk)
ISBN 0-7619-4180-0 (pbk)
© Glen Laverack 2004
First published 2004
Reprinted 2004, 2005

SAGE Publications Ltd
1 Oliver's Yard
55 City Road
London EC1Y 1SP

SAGE Publications Inc
2455 Teller Road
Thousand Oaks
California 91320

SAGE Publications India Pvt Ltd
B-42 Panchsheel Enclave
PO Box 4109
New Delhi – 100 017

British Library Cataloguing in Publication Data
A catalogue record for this book is available from the British Library

Library of Congress Control Number: 2003106175

Typeset by C&M Digitals Ltd., Chennai, India
Printed and bound in Great Britain by
Biddles Ltd, King's Lynn, Norfolk

Contents

List of Figures, Tables and Boxes

Figures

Tables

Boxes

Foreword

Most of us know that our health is more than good medical care when we are sick, or healthy living to stave off disease. Our daily lives teach us that our health is enwrapped in our experiences of community – a word that means 'the quality of sharing and caring' – and in our powers of choice, what Nobel economist Amartya Sen[1] calls our 'capacity to live a life one has reason to value'. Research increasingly affirms that social justice ('sharing'), social capital ('caring') and empowerment ('the capacity of choice') are key determinants of our health: as individuals, as communities, as societies. Power and the means to its attainment – empowerment – are what lies at the heart of this book.

For almost 30 years, a small practice within many countries' health sector has been acting upon this knowledge. Health promotion – a return to the public health activism of earlier centuries – describes the efforts of educators, social workers, nurses, physicians and other trained professionals (some of them even trained as 'health promoters') to give weight to that metric-adjusted truism of a gram of prevention being worth a kilogram of cure. For almost 30 years, its practice also has had to grapple with the seeming opposites it straddles. Is health promotion about changing unhealthy lifestyles or unhealthy living conditions? Does it target individuals or attempt collective mobilization? Should it preach self-regulation 'do this, don't do that' or espouse empowerment (autonomy of choice)? Perhaps most importantly, does its practice strike the right balance between valued professional expertise and invaluable community wisdom? No-one working in the field is blind to these tensions. But rarely are these the foci of an introductory text.

Not so with this book. Glenn Laverack, drawing upon his own experiences and a masterful summary of some of the important footsteps he encourages readers to follow, makes 'power' and its transformation the central theme of health promotion practice. Each of its transformative junctures is illustrated with case studies from practice. But there are two things that make this book a unique contribution. First is his synthesis of empowerment's major 'domains'. Second is his elucidation of a framework for how health promoters can make empowerment goals a 'parallel track' that can begin to link health promotion's befuddling 'top down'/'bottom up' opposites. The question is no longer whether health promoters should spend their time urging people to exercise more (unhealthy lifestyles), or organizing people around anti-poverty campaigns (unhealthy living conditions); depending on the context, either or both can be important health promoting priorities. The question, instead, is how can health promoters, regardless of the *content* of their programme work, plan it to facilitate desired changes in community empowerment's domains?

Readers may not close this book's last page with a recipe for a social marketing campaign, group educational session, community mobilization strategy or any of the other techniques that fill up health promotion's toolbox. Texts on those there are aplenty. But what they will take away is the foundational idea that health promotion is not only an 'evidence-based' technical practice, but an activist commitment to social change; and a few beguilingly simple yet fundamentally transformative tools to help them translate that idea into action.

Ronald Labonte
Director, Saskatchewan Population Health
and Evaluation Research Unit,
Universities of Saskatchewan and Regina, Canada

---

[1]Sen, A. (1999) *Development as Freedom*. New York: Knopf.

Preface

I call this book *Health Promotion Practice: Power and Empowerment*. What I mean by this title is that power, the ability to create or resist change, is an important foundation for individual and community health. It provides people with the capacities to change their lives and their living conditions. People experience power in many different ways and health promotion is one potential means by which this experience might be enhanced. This book is written, with an international context in mind, for persons who are, or are considering becoming, health promoters and who have the potential to enhance the power of others.

Empowerment, the process by which people gain more power, is at the heart of the 'new' health promotion that has arisen since publication of the Ottawa Charter for Health Promotion in 1986. The Charter has helped to define this 'new' practice and states that 'health promotion is a process of enabling people to increase control over, and to improve, their health' (World Health Organisation, 1986). I call this 'enabling' practice 'empowerment' and its outcome 'community empowerment'. At the same time individuals accrue more power; in fact, this is essential to the process but it is as a community, or group, phenomenon that I am most interested in empowerment in this book.

For over a century, many governments, religious and non-governmental organizations have attempted to improve the power of relatively poor or marginalized groups. They called this 'community development' and although it was rarely undertaken for health purposes, it often had an indirect effect of making people healthier.

Community empowerment as a concept rose in the 1980s and began to supplant the term 'community development'. Its popularity fell in the 1990s, tarnished by overuse, misuse and poor definition, although it is the term I prefer to use in this book precisely because of the emphasis it places on 'power'. Many practitioners and researchers now use the term 'community capacity building' to describe the same goals and practices of community development and community empowerment. All three terms (community development, empowerment and capacity) convey that there is something very important in the nature and quality of our day-to-day relationships 'in community': in our neighbourhoods, our workplaces, our leisure activities and through our friendships. These relationships, and the social conditions in which they exist, define who we are as people and play an important role in determining individual and community health. A community's success in making these conditions healthier is affected by its ability to mobilize resources, organize actions and partici-pate in decision-making that shape the social and physical world in which it exists. An empowering approach to health promotion helps to improve these abilities. Detailing how health promotion might do this is the main theme of this book.

This book comes from personal experiences as much as from an analy-sis of the literature. My intent is to share some of this experience, sup-ported by the wider literature and my discussions over the past several years with many other health promoters.

Acknowledgements

I would like to acknowledge the many people with whom I have had the privilege of working and exchanging ideas in relation to this book. In particular I would like to thank Dr Ronald Labonte for his insightful contributions to the early draft. I would also like to thank Professor John Catford; Dr John Hubley; Professor Lawry St Ledger; Dr Nina Wallerstein; Dr Kevin Brown; Dr Susan Rifkin and Dr Pat Pridmore. And to my family, Elizabeth, Ben, Holly and Rebecca for their continued support and patience during the course of writing this book.

An Overview of the Book

This book has three main purposes:

1   To introduce the readers to health promotion practice as a political activity, one that attempts to get at the underlying social determinants of disease.
2   To help the readers understand the importance of power relations, and their transformation in health promotion practice.
3   To introduce the readers to a new methodology for planning, implementing and evaluating empowering health promotion programmes.

Chapter 1   Health Promotion in Context

In Chapter 1 I define and discuss two key concepts: health promotion and community empowerment in the context of political activism. I also identify practice tensions that underpin health promotion's efforts to be 'empowering'.

Chapter 2   Promoting Health: it all Depends on What we Mean by 'Health'

Health promotion is about improving people's lives and health. But what do we mean by 'health' and how do our interpretations influence the way we approach different health promotion strategies? Chapter 2 discusses three main discourses of health, provides a simple framework of health determinants and explains their implication for an empowering health promotion practice.

Chapter 3   Power Transformation and Health Promotion Practice

Chapter 3 moves the reader into the territory of power, a concept that is central to the 'new' health promotion. But what does power look like and how can health promoters act to transform unhealthy into healthy personal and social power relationships? Chapter 3 addresses these questions and this allows conclusions to be reached about power and empowerment within health promotion practice in a programme context.

Chapter 4   Community Empowerment and Health Promotion Practice

In Chapter 4 I continue the discussion of power transformation and discuss the concept of community empowerment and how it can be successfully applied to health promotion practice to provide a more empowering approach.

Chapter 5   Addressing the Tensions in Health Promotion Programming

Chapter 5 extends the discussion of power and empowerment into the territory of health promotion programming. One of the basic tensions in an empowering health promotion practice is between 'top-down' approaches (in which experts decide what is best for communities) and 'bottom-up' approaches (in which communities work with experts on issues they both believe are important). I argue that these two approaches, and the power 'tensions' that they create, are not, or at least do not have to be, mutually exclusive.

Chapter 6   'Parallel-tracking' Community Empowerment into Health Promotion Programming

All health promotion work involves 'programmes', but not all ways of planning, implementing and evaluating programmes are empowering. Chapter 6 identifies the key differences and presents a framework for the systematic accommodation of community empowerment ('bottom-up' approaches) into 'top-down' health promotion programming.

Chapter 7   The Domains of Community Empowerment

Chapter 7 defines and describes the nine operational domains of community empowerment: participation; leadership; organizational structures;

problem assessment; resource mobilization; asking why; links with others; the role of outside agents; and programme management. These domains represent those aspects of the process of community empower ment that allow individuals and groups to organize and mobilize themselves toward social and political change, and they can be used to promote and evaluate this concept; discussed further in Chapters 8 and 9.

Chapter 8   Building Community Empowerment Approaches in Health Promotion

Chapter 8 provides two case study examples of empowering health promotion approaches that use the empowerment domains discussed in Chapter 7. A new methodology for building community empowerment is discussed and a case study of its successful implementation in Fiji is examined.

Chapter 9   Evaluating Community Empowerment Approaches

Chapter 9 addresses how we plan our health promotion programmes so that they will succeed in the evaluation of empowerment. These are important aspects of our work, not only for our employers (who need results to keep us employed), but also for our communities (is our work helpful to them?) and ourselves (how can we improve our efforts?). I discuss what to look for, and what evaluation methods to choose that are both rigorous and that fit with contemporary health promotion practice.

Chapter 10   Implications for an Empowering Health Promotion Practice

In the final chapter I discuss the broader implications and limitations for an empowering professional practice and examine the influence that the external context can place on practice, in particular the political, economic and socio-cultural contexts. I draw hope from the optimism that exists in health promotion practice, and examine how the organizational context in which health promotion practitioners work can provide more scope and opportunity to embrace empowerment.

1 Health Promotion in Context

John McKnight (1987), an influential American community health thinker, once observed that 'Universities learn by studies, institutions learn by reports and communities learn by stories'. While the distinction between these three approaches to knowledge is more blurred than we might think, the experiences from people's lives remain one of the most potent ways we have devised to share wisdom. Listening to the testimony of community members' experiences is also a basic starting point in the approach to health promotion used in this book. A story, then, seems an apt way to introduce some of the 'empowering' practice characteristics of health promotion, and the personal commitments it demands.

Health professional as political activist

In 1847, the Prussian province of Silesia was ravaged by a typhoid epidemic. Because the crisis threatened the population of coal miners in the area, and thus the economy, the Prussian government hired a young pathologist, Rudolf Virchow, to investigate the problem. His employers imagined that Virchow would return with the recommendation then in vogue: a little more fresh air, a little more fresh drinking water. But Virchow had much more to say about the situation.

He had spent three weeks in early 1848, not studying disembodied statistics or bureaucratic reports, but living with the miners and their families. One of the first points he made in his report to the Prussian government was that typhoid was only one of several diseases afflicting the coal miners, prime amongst the others being dysentery, measles and tuberculosis. Virchow referred to these diseases as 'artificial' to emphasize that, while they had their origin with a particular and 'naturally' occurring bacterium, their epidemic rates in Silesia were determined by poor housing, working conditions, diet and lack of sanitation amongst the coal miners. For Virchow, the answer to the question as to how to prevent typhoid outbreaks in Silesia was to incite the population to a united effort. Education, freedom and welfare would be attained only from the people's realization of their real needs.

To facilitate people realizing their own needs, Virchow proposed a joint committee involving both lay people and professionals. This group would monitor the spread of typhoid and other diseases while organizing agricultural food cooperatives to ensure that the people had sufficient food to eat. Virchow's solutions to the typhoid epidemic over the longer term, based on his talks with the miners and their families, were even more radical, and included improved occupational health and safety, better wages, decreased working hours and strong local and regional self-government. Virchow argued for progressive tax reform, removing the burden from the working poor and placing it on the *nouveau riche*, who expropriated great wealth from the mines while regarding the Silesians themselves not as human beings but as machines. He also advocated democratic forms of industrial development, and even suggested hiring temporarily unemployed miners to build roadways, making it easier to transport fresh produce during the winter.

These recommendations were not exactly what the Prussian government had expected. They had not hired Virchow to call into question the economics of the coal industry and industrial capitalism. He had none of the legitimating rhetoric of the Ottawa Charter for Health Promotion and its argument that health sectors needed to attend more to such 'basic health prerequisites' as 'peace, shelter, education, food, income, a stable ecosystem, social justice and equity' (World Health Organisation, 1986). Virchow was thanked for his report and promptly fired.

Scarcely one week later, on his return to Berlin, Virchow joined with other street demonstrators erecting barricades and demonstrating passionately for political changes that they hoped would bring democracy, which Virchow believed was essential for health. He established a radical, yet prestigious, magazine entitled *Medical Reform*, in which writers commented on the importance of full employment, adequate income, housing and nutrition in creating health. A decade later, still believing that political action was necessary for health, Virchow became a member of the Berlin Municipal Council and eventually of the Prussian Parliament itself. Throughout his 20 years as an elected official, Virchow campaigned tirelessly to get disease treated as a social as well as a medical issue. He planned and implemented a system of sewage disposal in Berlin and drafted legislation for proper food handling and inspection. He established better systems of building ventilation and heating, and introduced the first health service and health education programmes in the schools. He also lobbied to improve the working conditions of health professionals, particularly those of nurses.

To Virchow, there was no distinction between being a health professional and a political activist because all disease had two causes, one pathological and the other political. While he is largely remembered in medical schools for his enormous contributions to pathology, Virchow died believing that his most important work was the time he spent with the Silesian miners, understanding how social conditions can either create health or produce illness. That this story is from the past also allows us to see that our current interest in the social dimensions of health is not something new, rather something rediscovered (Taylor and Rieger, 1985).

Lessons from the past

Many diseases that consume us today, at least in more affluent countries, are different from the infectious ills of Virchow's time. But Virchow's story tells us that, whether infectious or chronic, diseases are physiological events that arise within, and derive their meaning, or significance, from particular social and political contexts.

Virchow's story also foreshadows the important role played by educated, empowered and organized groups of citizens in creating healthy social change. Infectious diseases declined dramatically in industrialized countries at the end of the last century, a transition in large part resulting from social and political changes:

- *Improved sanitation*. Many life-threatening infectious diseases such as cholera are spread through the contamination of drinking water by infected human sewage. Once sewage disposal was separate from sources of drinking water, water-borne diseases began to be reduced.
- *Improved working and living conditions*. Nineteenth-century factories were dirty and dangerous places to work. The clogged and smoggy air in the metal, textile and pottery towns damaged people's lungs and made them more susceptible to tuberculosis, one of the big killers of the past century. As occupational standards were drafted and enforced, workers' health improved. Labour standards and collective bargaining gradually raised workers' wages, shortened working weeks and eliminated child labour, while public education and more effective town planning improved social living conditions.
- *Improved nutrition*. As workers' wages improved, they could afford more nutritious foods, which strengthened their physical health and their abilities to resist infection.
- *Family planning*. The constant childbearing that was commonplace a hundred years ago literally wore out the bodies of many women. Not surprisingly, children who were born later into large families were weaker and more diseased than first-born children, reflecting the deteriorating conditions of their mother's bodies. With birth control and family planning came longer lived, healthier mothers, smaller families and less crowded living conditions.

These changes did not come easily. Employers often opposed sanitary reforms and quarantines on imported goods because they reduced profits. Working class organization for improved wages and better working conditions was often brutally repressed by élite groups whose interests were challenged. It can therefore be argued that many of the health gains of the nineteenth century arose from the entwined efforts of:

- organized workers' groups that struck for higher wages, safer conditions and the eight-hour day;

- organized women's groups that struggled for suffrage and the right to birth control;
- public health professionals, who lobbied for progressive social reforms and implemented sanitary and quarantine measures; and
- progressive political reformers, who wrote these claims for health and social justice in legislation.

Similar alliances are needed today for creating what is now called 'healthy public policies', or legislative reforms in environment, economy and social welfare that take into account their short and long term health implications. Even where the concerns are lifestyles, such as tobacco or alcohol abuse, the most dramatic and health-promoting changes have resulted from policy enactments governing product pricing and availability, or restrictions such as smoking bans in the workplace. These policy initiatives usually arise from partnerships between advocacy-oriented citizens' groups and public health professionals. When concern shifts from individual health behaviours to broader health conditions, such as poverty, inequality or discrimination, the role of community organizing and policy advocacy becomes even more important.

There are two other lessons for health promotion that can be taken from Virchow's story. First, Virchow was dismayed by how the poverty of the Silesian miners induced a sort of apathy or resignation and recognized that 'inciting the people to a united effort' is not easy work. While oppressed peoples often produce their own leaders and organizers, there is also an important 'outside' role that health promoters can play in this process. This role might include the specific knowledge, material and financial resources or organizing skills that the health promoter offers; for example, the health promoter represents a link between less powerful groups and more powerful public institutions, political and economic leaders. But central to this role is a motivational and power-transforming presence.

Second, Virchow's argument that the Silesian problem was not simply typhoid, but a whole range of diseases that shared in common an aetiology in people's living and working conditions, draws attention to a conundrum that still characterizes health promotion debate. Is it a practice intended to galvanize people into action around a specific set of risk factors associated with a specific disease? Or is it something larger and less easy to define that involves efforts by citizens, professionals and public institutions to make healthier, more deeply structured social conditions such as poverty, inequality and powerlessness? This raises important questions about evaluation and accountability; for example, Virchow's report on the plight of Silesian miners fell on deaf political ears. Does that mean his work failed? Or, to the extent that it played some small part in motivating new forms of organization amongst the miners, did his work provide political reformers with a potent health argument for their work and serve as an inspiration for public health activists? Might we then as easily conclude that Virchow's work succeeded? In other words, the process of empowerment that is central to health promotion change can be as important a success as the change itself.

What is health promotion?

Health promotion is not a new idea, if one takes it to mean any or all activities that improve the health of individuals and communities. Health promotion as a named practice, however, is more recent, with its steady rise in the health sectors of most industrialized countries following Canada's landmark 1974 publication *A New Perspective on the Health of Canadians* (Lalonde, 1974). Following in the tradition of earlier public health measures to curb the spread of infectious diseases, health promotion emphasized the importance of interventions to prevent disease and promote wellbeing rather than relying upon remedial efforts to treat their damaging effects. This emphasis, given the deliberate contrast many of its proponents make to costly medical care, has helped to make health promotion politically legitimate (World Health Organisation, 2002c). Despite its legitimacy, there remains a lot of disagreement amongst writers and practitioners about what health promotion 'really is'. These disagreements are illustrated by the three short stories in Box 1.1.

Box 1.1: Three faces of health promotion

Story 1: Sharon the nurse educator

Sharon is a nurse educator in a large teaching hospital. She runs groups for people who have been treated for serious heart disease. The goal of her education is to help people understand the importance of compliance with follow-up care (drugs, return check-ups) and the value of changing certain lifestyles (smoking, diet, exercise). Patients (which is how she thinks of them) are in the programme for as long as they are under formal hospital care. Success for her is an indication that the patients will comply with their treatment, that they have made an appointment with a local health centre after discharge and that, as Sharon puts it, 'They've had some fun in the group, since fun is a great healer.'

Story 2: Bob the nutritionist

Bob works for a local health department running nutrition and physical activity programmes tailored to low-income groups. Holding an advanced health promotion university degree, he appreciates the need for careful planning of his programmes: goals, objectives, activities, measurable and time-specific outcomes. He also appreciates the importance of a 'multifaceted' approach to health promotion. He supplements his education groups with some personal lobbying to make physical activity centres free to people on low incomes. His big concern is intervening early into, even preventing the onset of, diabetes, which his reading tells him is on the cusp of becoming a major epidemic amongst 'high risk' groups.

Story 3: Jill the social worker

Jill, a social worker by training, is part of a community health team employed by a local Health Trust. The Trust serves a severely disadvantaged area. A group was formed around timely access to health services and lack of safety and maintenance in the council housing. Jill was a key organizing resource in their work. She is attempting to get the group formalized in structure, and better linked to outside groups and other agencies that will add more political weight to their efforts. She has also formed a local chapter of the recently created Equity in Health Society and has published a few articles on her community empowerment approach to health promotion in practitioner journals.

In practice, the people in all three stories are right in claiming that they are doing health promotion. Health promotion is an idea that still belongs primarily to people employed in the health sector, in the sense that it provides these workers with some conceptual models, professional legitimacy and programmatic resources. Some of these workers may be titled 'health promoters' or 'community developers', others 'health educators', while many more who look to the idea of health promotion occupy more traditional job roles such as nurses, health visitors, physicians and social workers.

What the three stories also illustrate is that health promotion is best thought of as a 'situated practice' rather than as some universal theory of or approach to health. By this I mean that people, largely employed by (situated in) state agencies or state-funded non-governmental organizations (NGOs), engage in activities or programmes that are intended to improve or maintain the health of individuals and groups. Increasingly, such activities are undertaken with the cooperation of these groups and in collaboration with persons working in other sectors, both public and private. To a lesser extent, activities have broadened to include changing public policies that condition individual or group choices and behaviours, for example, pricing mechanisms to reduce tobacco consumption or new regulations to make housing healthier.

In broad terms, health promotion describes a relationship between the state (which regulates health opportunities), market economies (which create both health opportunities and health hazards) and community groups (which, through individual choices or collective action, influence both the state and market economies as well as their own health). More particularly, health promotion works to create some change in that relationship. This change could be defined as increasing citizen compliance with state health advice on fitness activities. Or it could be defined as improving the ability of marginalized groups to voice their concerns and influence political decision-making. By considering health promotion as a 'situated practice', our concern shifts away from any one particular health goal or target to the role of health promoters in making a valuable contribution to the attainment of that goal. Sharon, Bob and Jill all want to change people's health. But if we commit to the idea that health promotion is about increasing people's control over their health, we need to pay attention to how they define their own health goals, and how we, as practitioners, contribute to their goal attainment. This brings us to consider two variations in contemporary health promotion theory and practice.

Health promotion: two variations on a theme

If the single theme of health promotion is ensuring that people enjoy better health, there are two main variations in how theorists and practitioners interpret it. Andrew Tannahill (1985), a leading UK health promotion theorist, provides the term's more conventional usage as 'a realm of health-enhancing activities which differ in focus from currently dominant "curative", "high technology" or "acute" health services'. Like many others, Tannahill favours a precise definition of health promotion, one that emphasizes the importance of health authorities rationally planning for health needs 'objectively' determined through epidemiological study. In practice, this corresponds most closely with our first and second stories, the disease-specific or lifestyle change approach to health that Sharon and Bob undertake. This health promotion variation, though helpful for its emphasis on planning, has been criticized for failing to account for more structurally determined health risks, such as economic inequalities, environmental degradation or social discriminations, or for quality of life outcomes not captured when relying upon morbidity and mortality rates alone.

The second variation represents the direction in which health promotion has been slowly moving over the past 20 years, and is closer to Jill's work on housing as an underlying health determinant. But, just as the first variation has its critics, so does the second, particularly for its tendency to oppose medical and social explanations of illness, to focus on the future rather than the present, and to fail to take account of known processes of behaviour change. In Chapter 2 I will argue, and illustrate, that distinctions between the medical/behavioural and the social approaches to health promotion are helpful for analysis, but are much more blurred in practice. The second variation considers health promotion to be a more open and contested term that partly represents the health system's response to the 'knowledge challenges' of progressive social movements, such as women's rights, social justice and civil rights (anti-racist) of the past two decades.

I will now clarify the role of two issues that are important to our understanding of health promotion – social movements and health education – before discussing community empowerment.

Health promotion and New Social Movement Theory

Health promotion has been described as a social movement and the term 'new health promotion movement' is widely used in the literature (Minkler, 1989; Stevenson and Burke, 1991; Labonte, 1993; Robertson and Minkler, 1994). Robertson and Minkler (1994) have accredited the 'new health promotion movement' to a fundamental shift in the ways in which many professionals think, talk and write about health. The term is often discussed in the context of the discourse of social movements (Labonte, 1996, describes the term 'discourse' as an inter-related system of statements around commonly understood meanings and values resulting themselves from social factors and the interplay of power relations, rather than an individual's own ideas or beliefs) and is misleading because it hides the bureaucratic and sometimes controlling nature of health promotion towards civil society. To explain this I argue below that although health promotion is not itself a social movement, it does share the emancipatory discourse of New Social Movement Theory (NSMT).

Social movements cover a wide range of subjects such as gay rights, human rights, anti-nuclear and environmental issues, pressure groups, mass parties and social clubs. Social movements do have a structure, a pattern of inter-relations between individuals and groups, but this pattern evolves through its processes of mobilization, participation and organization. Formal social movements may possess bureaucratic procedures but they do not operate from within the bureaucracy. Social movements exist within civil society, developed by the people, against systematic structures and ideologies held by those in authority (Pakulski, 1991).

The main themes of the discourse of NSMT is the enhancement of control of civil society, democratization of the state, equity and social justice. The characteristic features of the NSMT are an emphasis on the anti-state/governance and its location which is placed very much within civil society. The New Social Movements, according to their theorists, have a fluid and dysfunctional nature shown by the disregard for social functions, often with no formal membership or programmes and ideologies which are expressed openly in public debate. Writing structured by the NSMT position tends to regard movements as essentially heterogeneous while displaying certain common characteristics such as scepticism against ideological blueprints, reformist orientations and self-limitation. This can result in the political goals of New Social Movements becoming self-limiting because they do not aim to seize state or economic power but instead challenge the dominant assumptions about knowledge and power (Melucci, 1989).

NSMT has an emancipatory role and places an emphasis on challenges to counter oppressive forms of power-over (discussed in Chapter 3) and the dominant discourse that has been taken for granted, created whilst gaining political legitimacy (Eyerman and Jamison, 1991). Examples of this is the environmental movement which challenged the knowledge that global resources were infinite, and the women's movement that challenged social stereotypes about gender roles, violence and rape. Various other rights movements have also challenged the dominant knowledge that shapes the way in which we think; for example, the gay, human and racial rights movements.

The main discourse of the NSMT is emancipation and social justice. Health promotion, in turn, uses a discourse which appeals for the empowerment of individuals and communities to enable them to take more control of decisions that influence their lives and health. The legitimization of this discourse came through the absorption of movement 'intellectuals' into government, academic and NGO positions (Eyerman and Jamison, 1991), and could be said to have been first codified by the Ottawa Charter for Health Promotion and by subsequent key international declarations (see Box 1.2).

Whilst health promotion shares the empowering and emancipatory discourse of NSMT, in practice it is often carried out within the controlling sphere of bureaucracy and of rational planning and accountability frameworks. Health promotion is not a social movement, but as Stevenson and Burke baldly state '... is a bureaucratic tendency, not a movement against the state, but one within it' (1991, p. 282).

Health promotion and health education

Health promotion is a contested term and whilst I have so far described it in terms of its practical application, there is no clear, widely accepted definition. In this book I generally adopt the World Health Organisation's (WHO) definition as a 'process of enabling people to increase control over, and to improve, their health' (World Health Organisation, 1986), which has its roots in the concept of individual and collective (community) empowerment, as I discuss later in this Chapter.

The debate about the overlap between health promotion and health education began in the 1980s when the range of activities involved in promoting better health widened to overcome the narrow focus on lifestyle approaches and the tendency to 'victim-blame' individuals for unhealthy behaviours. I discuss this in more detail in Chapter 2. These activities involved more than just giving information used in traditional health education and aimed for strategies that achieved political action, social mobilization and advocacy.

Keith Tones, an influential British health promotion commentator, and his colleagues (1990) suggest that health education and health promotion have a symbiotic relationship. Health education provides the agenda setting and critical consciousness raising in health promotion programmes. Without the inclusion of education strategies, health promotion programmes would be little more than manipulative processes of social coercion and community control. But, whereas health education is aimed at informing people to influence their future individual or collective decision-making, health promotion aims at complementary social and political actions, such as advocacy and community development, that facilitate political changes in people's social, workplace and community environments to enhance health (Green and Kreuter, 1991). Thus, health education around tobacco issues might include school-based awareness programmes or smoking cessation courses. Health promotion around tobacco issues extends to legislation restricting access to tobacco products, bans on advertising, and laws or policies restricting where smoking might be allowed.

Health promotion encompasses health education and I agree with the authors Linda Ewles and Ina Simnett (1999) that the most practical way forward is to view it as an umbrella term for a range of educational and health promoting activities.

Box 1.2: Key international health promotion declarations

Several international health promotion declarations have helped to define and legitimize new approaches to health promotion practice. These include:

The 1978 Declaration of Alma Ata (World Health Organisation, 1978) recognized that the gross inequalities in the health status between and within countries were unacceptable, and identified primary health care as the key to attaining 'Health for All'. The Declaration pointed to the special needs for the promotion and protection of health in developing countries and that the spirit of development should be one of social justice towards world peace. The Declaration recognized that people must be actively involved in the process of development and states: 'The people have the right and duty to participate individually and collectively in the planning and implementation of their health care.' The Declaration goes beyond simply increased participation to imply that empowerment is a necessary component of primary health care.

The 1986 Ottawa Charter for Health Promotion (World Health Organisation, 1986) identified a number of prerequisites or fundamental conditions and resources which are crucial for the improvement of health: peace, shelter, education, food, income, a stable eco-system, sustainable resources, social justice and equity. The Charter thus expanded the outcomes for health promotion beyond the absence of disease or the adoption of healthy lifestyles. The Charter defined five health promotion action areas for achieving better health.

1 Building healthy public policy.
2 Creating supportive environments.
3 Strengthening community action.
4 Developing personal skills.
5 Re-orienting health services.

It also described three important roles for health promoters – advocating, enabling and mediating – and became the founding document of the 'new' health promotion movement.

The 1988 Adelaide Conference Statement (World Health Organisation, 2002a) addressed the first of the five action areas, building healthy public policy. The conference statement endorsed the Declaration of Alma Ata and stated that 'health is both a fundamental human right and a sound social investment'. It went on to state that '… inequalities in health are rooted in inequalities in society. Closing the health gap would require public policy that improved access to health enhancing goods and services and created supportive environments.'

The 1991 Sunsdvall Conference Statement (World Health Organisation, 2002b) was the first WHO health promotion conference to have a global perspective, with participants from 81 countries. This conference addressed the second of the five action areas for health promotion, creating supportive environments. This encompasses both the physical and social aspects of where people live, work and play. The conference highlighted four important aspects of supportive environments:

1 Traditional values and beliefs, customs, social processes and rituals that provide a sense of belonging, coherence and purpose.
2 Governmental commitment to human rights, social justice, peace and democracy.
3 Re-channelling economic resources into the achievement of 'Health for All' and away from the arms race.
4 The important role of women in creating supportive environments, and the need to stop their exploitation.

The 1997 Jakarta Conference Statement (World Health Organisation, 2002c) endorsed health as a basic human right, affirmed the five action areas of the Ottawa Charter and proposed (somewhat controversially) that new partnerships, especially with the private sector, were important to the success of health promotion. The Conference Declaration also affirmed that there is clear evidence that:

• comprehensive approaches to health development are the most effective;
• 'settings' (such as families, neighbourhoods, communities) for health offer practical opportunities for the implementation of comprehensive strategies;

- participation by all people is essential to sustain efforts;
- health literacy fosters participation; and
- access to education and information is essential to achieving effective participation and the empowerment of people and communities.

The 2000 Mexico Global Conference for Health Promotion (World Health Organisation, 2002d) sought to demonstrate how health promotion strategies add value to the effectiveness of health and development policies, programmes and projects, particularly those that aim to improve the health and quality of life of people living in adverse circumstances. The Conference Statement recognized that health is not only an outcome of, but also an important input into, economic development and equity. It also declared that health promotion and social development 'is a central duty and responsibility of governments' and that 'health promotion must be a fundamental component of public policies and programmes in all countries in the pursuit of equity and better health for all'. The Conference also challenged health promotion to pay closer attention to global phenomena, such as the re-appearance and broader spread of the HIV/AIDS pandemic in Africa and growing global disparities in wealth and health.

What is community empowerment?

The WHO's definition of health promotion as 'increasing people's control over their health' places it alongside our other key concept: community empowerment. Community empowerment has different conceptual roots from health promotion, arising primarily from international development work (poor communities needed to become more powerful), the women's health movement (which challenged the prerogative of then usually male doctors to define women's health concerns and remedies) and community mental health activists (who stressed that people with mental disease deserved similar rights to others and ought to be treated in 'empowering' rather than controlling ways).

Community empowerment can be viewed as both a process (something used to accomplish a particular goal or objective) and an outcome (in which empowerment is the goal or objective itself). In this book I view community empowerment as both and define it as an interactive process moving in either direction along a continuum involving personal empowerment, the development of small mutual support groups, community organizations and networks or coalitions (Labonte, 1990; Rissel, 1994). The outcome of empowerment will be specific to the individual, group or community involved, although there is also a general goal, similar to how the Ottawa Charter defines health promotion: that people involved in the empowerment process gain more control over important decisions and social structures that influence their lives. This often leads to collective social and political action. Consequently, the outcomes of community empowerment can have a very long time frame (Raeburn, 1993), often taking several years to begin to show results.

There is considerable overlap between community empowerment and other concepts such as community participation (Rifkin, 1990), community capacity building (Goodman et al., 1998), community competence (Eng and Parker, 1994) and community development (Labonte, 1998). They describe a process that increases the assets and attributes which a community is able to draw upon in order to improve their lives (including, but not restricted to, their health). The concepts are also fundamentally addressing the same thing: new forms of social organization and collective action to redress the inequalities in the distribution of power (decision-making authority) and resources. This is important for health promoters because a great deal of our health is determined by the power that we experience and our control over resources. In this book I use community empowerment to describe the process by which communities (and the individuals within them) gain more control, and community capacity as the domains or specific attributes through which that control is exercised.

In a westernized context community empowerment is often seen in individualistic terms, as '… a raised level of psychological empowerment among its members, a political action component in which members have actively participated, and the achievement of some redistribution of resources or decision making favourable to the community in question' (Rissel, 1994). Community empowerment builds from the individual to the group to the broader community. In non-westernized countries empowerment can take on a very different interpretation, not as an individual or solitary phenomenon but one that is more closely connected to the family or extended kin systems (Erzinger, 1994). In a traditional Fijian context I found that the concepts of power and empowerment were closely connected to chieftaincy and community leadership (Laverack, 1998). Community empowerment builds from these family networks to the broader community. It is always important that we check our interpretation of empowerment to ensure it is relevant to the cultural context of the people involved in our health promotion programmes.

Health promotion programming: it's all about power transformation

In this book I intend to show how the two main health promotion variations (a focus on health behaviour programmes and a commitment to healthy social change in underlying conditions) can and should work together as one. The empowerment variation, embedded in the Ottawa Charter, has proved difficult to put into practice, and many health promoters find themselves torn between the 'top-down' approach of lifestyle disease prevention programmes and 'bottom-up' community empowerment projects. Part of the problem lies with the health authorities and NGOs who employ health promoters, and who are often nervous of the less easily controlled and more political aspects of community empowerment. Part of the problem also lies in health promoters themselves, who often have a superficial understanding of the meaning of power, lack clarity about the influences on the process of community empowerment, or do not have a clear understanding of how community empowerment can be practically accommodated within health promotion practice.

Julian Rappaport (1985), the principal empowerment theorist from the community mental health stream, argues that empowerment cannot be given; those who seek it must take it. Those that have power or have access to it, such as health promoters, and those who want it, such as the community members, must work together to create the necessary conditions to make empowerment possible. Theories of power are discussed in Chapter 3. The challenge for health promoters is how these necessary conditions might be made possible in health promotion programming.

Health promotion programmes predominantly use two seemingly different approaches that I have characterized as 'top-down' and 'bottom-up'. The distinguishing characteristic between these two approaches is who determines the issue being addressed by the programme.

In conventional top-down programming the outside agents (such as a government department or NGO) define the issue, develop strategies to resolve the issue and involve the community to assist in implementing the strategies. The objectives and design of the programme are predetermined and are usually concerned with specific targets, using quantifiable indicators. Not surprisingly, some health promotion commentators (Boutilier, 1993) argue that these types of programmes contradict the spirit, if not also the principles, of the Ottawa Charter for Health Promotion. These programmes generally focus on a negative definition of health, such as the need to prevent cancer or heart disease, and are concerned primarily with lifestyle and behavioural compliance to certain professionally determined norms. Some well-known examples of top-down health promotion programmes are the Multiple Risk Factors Intervention Trial (MRFIT), the Community Intervention Trials for Smoking Cessation (COMMIT) and the North Karelia Project on cardiovascular disease (discussed in Chapter 5).

In bottom-up programming the outside agents act to support the community in the identification of issues which are important and relevant to their lives, and to enable them to develop strategies to resolve these issues. The programme design and management is negotiated with the community, there is a longer and more loosely defined time frame and the programme is often explicitly concerned with the process of empowerment and capacity building. Health promoters have conventionally viewed community empowerment as a part of bottom-up approaches.

Few health promotion programmes adopt a purely bottom-up approach (Canadian Public Health Association, 1996; Labonte, 1998). The same design characteristics that provide evidence of the success of bottom-up programmes, a long time frame, small size, and the control by community members, primarily appear to be those which make them unattractive to many outside agents. But while it is true that most health promoters orient their work towards a top-down, disease prevention and lifestyle approach, others are passionately engaged in bottom-up, community development initiatives around such issues as poverty, violence and housing. More importantly, the two approaches are better thought of as ideal types of theoretical usefulness rather than hard-and-fast approaches to practice. The dichotomy between top-down disease prevention and lifestyle change and bottom-up community empowerment approaches is not as fixed as it is sometimes portrayed. Many health promoters, in their community work, shift between the options of marketing and managing lifestyle programmes and efforts to organize and support community efforts to change health risks in their physical and social environments. Health authorities may still keep considerable control and may not act upon all the issues raised by the community, but the priorities are no longer the same as would be if the programme used a singularly top-down approach.

The challenge for health promoters becomes how they can include the concerns and issues of the community in top-down programming. To help meet this challenge, in Chapter 6 I show how the process of community empowerment can be viewed as a 'parallel track' running alongside the main 'programme track'. I describe this as an 'empowering approach' where capacity-building is the process used to develop more empowered and capable communities. Community empowerment is sometimes seen as the means to an end: health promoters want to build capacity so that communities are better able to comply with or sustain the health promotion programme. I take this further and describe how health promotion programmes can also be seen as a means to building community empowerment/capacity. At issue is how the programme and the empowerment tracks become linked during the progressive stages of the top-down programme cycle.

I begin, in Chapter 2, by exploring the different ways in which people define 'health', and its implications for health promotion. I also discuss a simple framework to explain the determinants of health and discuss the challenges this poses for an empowering health promotion practice.

2 Promoting Health: it all Depends on What we Mean by 'Health'

Health promotion is about improving people's lives and health. But what do we mean by 'health'? There are many different ways to define health, each of them leading to different health promotion strategies. How we define and interpret health largely determines how we approach health promotion. This chapter discusses three main discourses of health and of health promotion and argues that a socio-environmental model of health is most consistent with health promotion's concern with empowerment. I also provide a simple framework of health determinants, and discuss its implication for an empowering health promotion practice.

Our experiences of health

When you ask people to talk about what is health in the abstract, they often reply 'Oh, not being sick, having no disease, keeping fit, not smoking, eating right'. These are the dominant discourses (defined in Chapter 1), or language-woven ways, of thinking about health. Health is portrayed in our culture as an aspect of physical breakdown or invasion (a medical problem) or the result of not heeding the proper lifestyle advice (a behavioural problem). But if you ask people to talk about the last time they felt healthy, when you personalize the question, quite different dimensions arise. They are more likely to talk about a sense of purpose in their lives, some control over their fate, doing enjoyable activities, feeling energetic and vital and, most of all, being loved, enjoying good relationships with friends, being connected to a 'community'.

Labonte (1993) asked participants of several workshops to 'Think of the last time you experienced yourself as "healthy", and jot down a few phrases that describe the feeling, and the context.' Few of the respondents were concerned with disease or ill health and instead identified feelings of 'energy', 'love', 'control', 'happy relationships', 'wholeness' and 'playfulness'. Box 2.1 collects a number of these phrases. Noticeably absent from this list is any reference to disease, and minimal attention is given to physical evaluations such as fitness levels.

Box 2.1: Experiences of health

energized
being loved, loving
being in control
fitting in, doing
relaxed, stress-free
giving/receiving, sharing
outdoors, nature
friends, belonging, meaning in life
able to do things I enjoy
peak physical shape
happiness, wholeness
spiritual contentment

(Labonte, 1993)

Health, the positive expression of our wellbeing, resides in the quality of sharing and caring in our relationships. The word 'health' derives from an old English word, hael, which brings us two other contemporary terms: whole and hello. The folk wisdom of our language posits health as intrinsically holistic. Our health systems may fragment hospitals into departments of particular body parts, or try to differentiate between diseases that are somatic (physical) and those which are psychological (mental). Our public systems may divide into services about health, education, environment or welfare. Our political and economic systems more generally may attempt to separate what is 'public' (government) from what is 'private' (market). But we do not experience our lives as discrete, disconnected events. Whether with friends, or physicians, we usually try to context whatever we experience physically with how we are feeling mentally, with self-judgements about our own behaviours and with some understanding of the role played by our broader living and working conditions.

The different definitions of health and their relation to health promotion practice is discussed in detail elsewhere (Downie et al., 1996; Dines and Cribb, 1993; Ewles and Simnett, 1999; Adams et al., 2002). Here I focus on the relevance of these definitions to the aspects of power and empowerment, the two central themes of this book.

Health, health promotion and social capital

In a fundamental way, our health is a reflection of the quality of our relationships with one another. Social support and network density reflect the language of social psychologists. Community psychologists might refer to the same phenomenon as 'community capacity', 'community competence' or 'community empowerment'. Political economists have recently coined the term 'social capital' to capture this caring and sharing dimension of our communal living. Putnam et al. (1993) have written widely and were early commentators on social capital and define it as the features of social organization such as networks, trust, facilitated coordination and collaboration. These are elements that are important to the process of community empowerment, discussed later in Chapter 4, by linking individuals to the groups and organizations that allow collective (community) action. Active participation within these social networks builds the trust and cohesiveness between individuals that are important to mobilize and create the resources necessary to support collective action.

Lee Adams, Mary Amos and James Munro (2002), three British health promoters, discuss the role of social capital in improving and sustaining health in three ways:

- by emphasizing the importance of social approaches to health promotion;
- by suggesting that social capital can act as a buffer against the worst effects of deprivation; and
- by focusing attention on the importance of social relationships and networks to community-based health efforts, for example through community empowerment, to reduce inequalities in health.

The notion of social capital suggests that inequalities in health are in part influenced by power imbalances in society and the ability of communities to empower themselves in redressing a lack of equity. By building community empowerment we can also build social capital. The risk is that the idea of building social capital may divert our attention away from the causes of inequality onto its effects, thus obscuring our analysis. Adams et al. (2002) also caution that our expectations of social capital in health promotion practice should be modest as many of the assumptions underpinning this concept, including its sustainability in a community context, need to be further examined. However, this does not invalidate the importance of community empowerment as an approach in health promotion practice.

The World Health Organisation's definition of health

The subjective or lay meanings people give to health does not imply that the term loses all precision in meaning. Cross-cultural studies indicate that people's experiences of health, such as those in Box 2.1, can usefully be organized under the following six broad categories:

1   Feeling vital, full of energy.
2   Having a sense of purpose in life.
3   Experiencing a connectedness to 'community'.
4   Being able to do things one enjoys.
5   Having good social relationships.
6   Experiencing a sense of control over one's life and one's living conditions.

(Blaxter, 1990; Labonte, 1993; 1998)

These six categories make sense of the World Health Organisation's classic definition of health as 'a state of complete physical, mental and social wellbeing, and not merely the absence of disease or infirmity.' Physical wellbeing is concerned with concepts such as the well functioning of the body, biological normality, physical fitness and capacity to perform tasks. Social wellbeing includes interpersonal relationships as well as wider social issues such as marital satisfaction, employability and community involvement. The role of relations, the family and status at work are important to a person's social wellbeing. Mental wellbeing involves concepts such as self-efficacy, subjective wellbeing, social competence and psychological hardiness.

Terri Jackson, Sally Mitchell and Maria Wright (1989), three Australian commentators on community development, recount the story of how and by whom the WHO definition was written. It was written soon after the Second World War by a WHO official who had spent the War working in the Resistance. He had come to this definition from this experience and explained that he had never felt healthier than during that terrible period: for he daily worked for goals about which he cared passionately; he was certain that should he be killed in his dangerous work his family would be cared for by the network of Resistance workers. It was under these circumstances that he felt most healthy, most alive. The definition of health was originally developed by a person who was passionately involved with others to change social and political structures. In other words, they are involved in taking control over those things which affect their lives and by doing so empower themselves and improve their own health and wellbeing as well as that of others with whom they associate. Rootman and Raeburn (1994) provide a later account in which the definition seems to have arisen originally as a medical solution to the ills of the world, as seen immediately post-War, the irony being that the definition is now so often seen as liberating health from the thrall of the medical model and definition.

Whatever its origins, the WHO conceptualization of health as an ideal state of physical, social and mental wellbeing that enables people to fulfil their health has been thoroughly cross-examined and criticized for not taking other dimensions of health into account, namely the emotional, spiritual and societal aspects of health. The definition has also been criticized for viewing health as a state or product rather than as a dynamic relationship, a capacity, a potential or a process. But mostly the definition has been criticized for specifying an idealistic state that is impossible to attain (Aggleton, 1991).

People are not concerned if their health is perfect but instead are concerned with the trade-offs they have to make in order to gain their optimum health. Cohen and Henderson (1991: 3) cite examples of people who are diseased or ill and yet still perceive themselves as being healthy and willing to bear the discomfort and pain of an illness because it does not outweigh the inconvenience, loss of control or financial cost of having the condition treated. These individuals undertake a cost–benefit analysis in regard to achieving optimum health 'where the cost of any further improvement outweighs the value attached to that improvement'. At an individual level, these are the 'positive' health outcomes to which health promotion programmes can contribute and have varying degrees of importance to people at different times in their lives. They are the 'trade-offs' people make in deciding what they need, or want to do, to experience being healthy.

Contemporary health approaches in health promotion

There are at least five established approaches to health promotion that are discussed in the literature: the medical approach; the behavioural approach; the educational approach; the client centred approach; and the socio-environmental approach. These are discussed elsewhere (Ewles and Simnett, 1999; Downie et al., 1996) and here I focus on three of the main contemporary approaches in health promotion – the medical, the behavioural and the socio-environmental – as being especially relevant to shaping the way in which we design, implement and evaluate programmes. For example, the medical approach views health as an absence of disease or disease-producing physiological conditions. The behavioural approach views health in terms of the behaviour and lifestyle of individuals, and the socio-environmental approach views health as being influenced by social and environmental conditions. These differing views largely determine the strategies programme planners select, and the outcomes or criteria they use to evaluate success. The development of these approaches in recent decades has resulted not only from the changes in our scientific understanding of health determinants and risk factors, but also from a growing pressure from individuals, groups and social movements concerned with the health impacts of social and environmental conditions.

The medical approach

Despite the evolution of competing health approaches, it is the medical approach that remains dominant, socially and within health bureaucracies.

This approach evolved as a result of scientific discoveries and technological advances in the eighteenth and nineteenth centuries and a greater understanding of the structure and functioning of the human body. As knowledge and understanding increased, the body became viewed as a machine that needed to be fixed. A professional split between the body and mind developed; the body and its physical illness was the responsibility of physicians, while psychologists and psychiatrists looked after the condition of the psyche. The focus remained on the external causes of ill health and was reinforced by the constant threat of disease and death, particularly to children, from epidemics such as polio and scarlet fever. The medical profession established itself in the dominant position, and many other health professions modelled themselves on the medical approach to gain legitimacy. These include the fields of nursing, physiotherapy and, until recently, health promotion (Baum, 1990).

The medical approach is primarily concerned with the absence of disease and the treatment of illness. More recently it has become concerned with disease prevention amongst high-risk individuals, those persons whose genetic pre-disposition, behaviour or family and personal history place them at statistically greater risk of disease. The medical approach historically has assumed that élite 'experts' know best. Disease prevention programmes in the medical approach are usually delivered in a top-down approach based upon the experts' knowledge. However, a growing body of new knowledge and pressure from social movements challenged the dominance of the medical approach. By the 1970s this had led to a broadening of health knowledge to include a variety of behavioural, lifestyle and social factors.

The behavioural/lifestyle approach

Lifestyle and behaviours became increasingly central to health promotion in the 1970s. During this period, health promoters (though many still called themselves health educators) recognized that individuals' behaviours and lifestyle could directly influence their own health and the health of others. Examples of programmes from this era include school education, public education and social marketing campaigns around smoking, alcohol abuse, eating high-fat foods, not wearing a seat belt and physical inactivity. The predominant approach to address these issues was education and awareness campaigns to inform individuals about their high-risk behaviours.

Given the complex social and cultural circumstances associated with lifestyle, it is not surprising that many practitioners and researchers found that health education campaigns alone did not succeed very much in changing behaviour.

The lifestyle approach does not necessarily view behaviour as an isolated action under the autonomous control of the individual, but recognizes how it is influenced and conditioned by a complex interplay of social, political and cultural factors. Much of the health promotion work under the lifestyle approach, however, continues to be on individuals rather than on their context. Meredith Minkler (1989) argues that this is because many health promoters are embedded in both western and uniquely American value systems, which place strong emphasis on the responsibility of the individual and the importance of autonomy and personal achievement.

The socio-environmental approach

The lifestyle approach argued for a more comprehensive view to health promotion than simply health education about specific diseases (the medical approach). It presented health promoters with a complex interplay of social and cultural factors that only the most ambitious, long term and complicated of programmes could hope to achieve (Green and Kreuter, 1991). At the same time, there was a growing professional frustration with health education and lifestyle approaches in health promotion because of the tendency to 'victim-blame' individuals by assuming that they were individually responsible for their own actions. The lifestyle approach failed to recognize the structural issues in which personal behaviours are embedded and which also indirectly but powerfully influence health, such as poverty. Inherent in the design of many of these programmes is a power-struggle between professional and client and between communities and health promotion organizations over who identifies or 'names' the health issue(s) to be addressed.

The critiques of the behavioural approach gained momentum during the late 1970s and early 1980s, stemming in part from the feminist, environmentalist and other social movements of this period. These social movements challenged the notion of the medical and behavioural approaches to health by raising concerns for social justice and environmental sustainability. The critiques argued that health, particularly of marginalized groups, was primarily influenced by structural issues such as poverty, housing, over-population and lack of community control. A new, emancipatory discourse on health promotion began to form, one more concerned with social justice and ecological sustainability than with individual behaviour change (see Box 2.2 for a brief discussion of two different, and important, ways of thinking about social justice).

> **Box 2.2: Health promotion and social justice: equality of opportunity or equality of outcome?**
>
> One of the major criticisms of the health promotion discourse as espoused by the Ottawa Charter is that it does not adequately address issues of social justice (Stevenson and Burke, 1991; Labonte, 1993; Canadian Public Health Association, 1996). Social justice has two different meanings. One is 'equality of opportunities', in which socio-political systems seek to maximize people's equal access to public resources and market opportunities, allowing them to experience satisfaction in their lives. The other meaning stresses 'equality of outcomes', in which socio-political systems seek to minimize serious and preventable inequalities between people. This requires a much more 'activist' state concerned with the equitable, or fair, distribution and re-distribution of resources. Don Nutbeam (1997: 14) defines equity in health as meaning '... that people's needs guide the distribution of opportunities for wellbeing'. This implies that people with greater needs, often because of poverty, discrimination or other forms of social exclusion, require and deserve greater opportunities. This is particularly so in developing countries, which often lack the resources taken for granted in richer countries. To move closer to equality in outcomes, including health outcomes, societies need to allow inequalities in opportunity that favour historically disadvantaged groups. For health promoters, this means taking care that those who benefit from their programmes or resources are not disproportionately the better-off. Instead, health promoters need to continue to give priority to groups whose poorer health is determined in large measure by their historically unequal opportunities.

The overlap between health promotion approaches

Table 2.1 below provides a summary of the different explanatory systems of the three health approaches. While each of these functions exists as a particular health discourse, shaping how practitioners go about their work, their distinctions often can and should blur. They are more like a Russian doll, one inside the other, than wholly separate ways of thinking. The medical approach, the most precise in definition, occupies the smallest doll. The behavioural approach incorporates the medical approach within a slightly larger doll that includes 'space' for individual behaviours and the social norms that shape them. The socio-environmental approach incorporates both the behavioural and the medical in the largest doll, whose new 'space' is cluttered with all of the social, economic and political structures that shape not only individual lifestyles but also people's risks of disease or opportunities for wellbeing.

Table 2.1 Three different health explanatory systems

	Medical	Behavioural	Socio-environmental
Health defined as:	biomedical, absence of disease, disability.	medical, plus functional ability, personal wellness, healthy lifestyles.	medical and behavioural, plus quality of life, social relationships.
Health explained by:	pathology, physiological risk factors.	medical, plus behavioural risk factors.	medical and behavioural plus psychosocial risk factors and socio-environmental risk conditions.
Target for intervention:	high risk individuals.	high risk groups.	high risk conditions.
Sample success criteria:	decreased morbidity, age standardized mortality, prevalence of physiological risk factors;	improved individual lifestyles (behaviour change);	improved social relationships and networks;
	improved individual QALYs.	adoption of healthier lifestyles earlier in 'lifecycle';	improved quality of life;
		decreased population physiological and behavioural risk factors.	movement towards social equity (more equal distribution of wealth/power);
			movement towards environmental sustainability.

Source: Labonte, 1993: 33–5.

Sharon, the nurse educator in Box 1.1, is quite right to be focused on people's ability to recover from a life-threatening, painful and often disabling medical event. But even she recognizes that the quality of social interaction amongst her group members is as important as the compliance lessons she is trying to teach them. She already stretches herself a little into the lifestyle approach by looking at their smoking or nutrition choices. But she needs to think further and deeper: what if the people she discharges return home to a house with inadequate insulation or plumbing? Or are members of a family with insufficient means to afford nutritious food? Or has an unemployed and depressed spouse been unable to offer any healing support? Unless these socio-environmental issues become part of how Sharon thinks and plans her work, chances are her patients will simply continue to return to her care with the same illnesses.

To a lesser extent the same applies to Bob in Box 1.1. He's already trying to create supportive environments to help make healthy choices (such as good food and exercise) the easy choices. But what if some of the diabetic women he's trying to help lack any child support or child care? What if a major fear for new migrants is walking in the evening to go to their local recreation centre because they might be attacked or threatened by people with racist attitudes? These are socio-environmental risk conditions that affect their personal choices, even when they know what to do, and want to do it.

As for Jill, her concern with the 'big health issues', such as equity in housing, risks leaving behind some of the very disadvantaged individuals she wants to help. Not every marginalized person wants to become an activist/advocate. Some are even quite concerned about their diets and their smoking, and wouldn't mind non-patronizing help in becoming personally healthier. People who are individually healthier are also better equipped, both physically and psychically, to take on the challenge of social activism.

The necessity to practice thinking through all three approaches at the same time becomes more obvious when we consider an analytical framework that illustrates how social inequalities become health inequities.

What determines health? An analytical framework of health determinants

David Seedhouse (1997), a former health promoter now health philosopher, has accused health promotion of being a 'magpie' profession. Like the bird's confusion of black and white splotches, health promotion lacks consistency in how it defines what it does, explains why it does it and how it accounts for its accomplishments. Seedhouse's point is that there often is inconsistency in how health promoters, and other public health practitioners, approach their work.

Part of this inconsistency derives from confusion over what health promotion seeks to promote: disease prevention, or positive health? But even if a useful model of positive health begins to supplant the 'death by disease' default model of most health systems, there are still two other questions that need answering. First, how are the more individualized experiences of positive health affected by social and environmental conditions? That is, what are the public health implications of positive health? Second, how do practitioners explain the important 'determinants' of health, those individual and social phenomena that comprise its territory of interest?

Several frameworks and models of health determinants now exist (for example, Evans and Stoddart, 1990; Dahlgren and Whitehead, 1992; Labonte, 1998; Starfield, 2001). The one offered in Figure 2.1 was originally developed for the federal Canadian Heart Health Initiative (Labonte, 1992) and the Toronto Health Department (Toronto Department of Public Health, 1991a) and has subsequently been adopted by the WHO. It is helpful to both

Figure 2.1   An analytical framework for the determinants of health

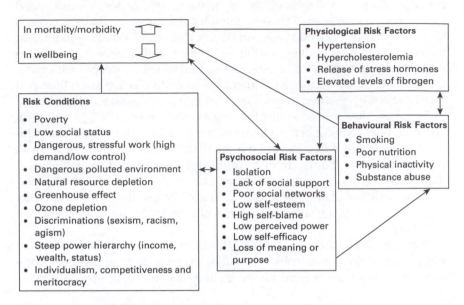

Source: Labonte 1993; 1998.

the students and practitioners of health promotion and addresses 'risk conditions', surplus powerlessness and learned helplessness, issues that are relevant to one of the core subjects of this book: power.

In summary, the argument this framework advances is that people living in risk conditions independently have more disease and premature death and less wellbeing. Risk conditions describe living and working conditions that are 'deeply structured' by economic and political practices, and by dominant ideologies or discourses. People often internalize the unfairness of their social circumstances as aspects of their own 'badness', thereby increasing their psychosocial risk factors, which are also associated with poorer health outcomes. All of this increases health-threatening physiological risk factors.

The analytical framework describes outcomes as wellbeing or positive health, and as mortality/morbidity. People who experience the risk conditions and risk factors described below are also less likely to report themselves as feeling healthy, or being happy, precisely because they lack the sense of control or capacity and the respectful social relationships that constitute people's experiences of wellbeing.

Risk conditions

The existence of risk conditions, or living and working conditions that, in Giddens's (1984) terms, are 'conditioned and constrained' by economic and political practices, increases disease risk and reduces wellbeing. Some of these conditions are universal and thus (more or less) equitable; for example, everyone suffers with ozone depletion. But most of these conditions are unequally distributed by virtue of being conditions of comparative inequality. One cannot have low status without someone else having high status. One cannot be poor without someone else being wealthy. The higher one's social status (one's power and wealth), the higher one's health status. The more steeply hierarchical this distribution of power and wealth, the greater the difference in health status between top and bottom (Evans et al., 1994; Smith, 1996; Wilkinson, 1996).

There is a huge literature on the effects of risk conditions such as poverty, social hierarchies and inequalities on health, both for individuals and for whole populations (Wilkinson, 1986; 1996). Deaths due to specific diseases and their individual risk factors change over time. Several decades ago, the poor died more frequently than the rich from infectious disease. Today, they die more frequently than the rich from heart disease, or from certain forms of cancer. Similarly, lower social class groups in different countries die from different causes (Smith et al., 1990). In England, they die more frequently from lung diseases and lung cancer. In France, they die more frequently from liver cirrhosis.

I do not attempt to review this literature, but use the framework in Figure 2.1 to demonstrate the effect that 'risk factors' have on health promotion practice and in particular on the role of power and empowerment.

Psychosocial risk factors

The pathways between oppression and unhappiness may be fairly obvious, but the links to disease are harder to identify. Research findings focus more on individuals than on populations, or what Figure 2.1 refers to as 'psychosocial risk factors'. This term describes individual cognitive or emotional states (such as self-esteem or self-blame) that are often reactions to risk conditions, and which also influence our desire and ability to create social networks and support systems. Health can be seen to be determined both by material conditions and relations (risk conditions), and by the meanings one makes of these psychosocial risk factors. Notably, how one comes to understand one's position in human hierarchies (Wilkinson, 1996) and the stress created by economic insecurity (lack of predictability over future employment/income). Occupational stress research finds that those workers with least predictability or control over their work suffer the greatest stress and its associated risks of heart disease. Lower status civil servants suffer disproportionate stress and disease consequent to the employment uncertainty introduced by such business practices as contracting out and down-sizing (Baum, 1990). The process by which structural inequality becomes physical pathology, then, might be described as follows: people living in risk conditions experience distress with the unfairness of their situation (their low status on some hierarchy of power or authority, indicated in part by wealth) and internalize this unfairness as aspects of their own 'badness' or 'failure'. This internalization adds to their distress, if not also to their loss of meaning and purpose, with measurable effects on their bodies such as hypertension and hypercholesterolemia, or what this model calls 'physiological risk factors'. This situation is more likely when the dominant social discourse on success is competitiveness, individualism and meritocracy, where people are presumed to succeed or fail purely on the basis of their own initiative or ability (Lerner, 1986).

This internalization of 'badness' leads to what philosophers describe as false consciousness, 'failing to utilize the power that one has and failing to acquire powers that one can acquire' (Morriss, 1987 p. 94), what psychologists call 'learned helplessness' (Seligman and Maier, 1967; Seligman, 1975), what political scientists label 'surplus powerlessness' (Lerner, 1986). More cynical commentators sometimes term this as the 'apathy of the poor'. Learned helplessness is a psychological construct that emerged from Martin Seligman's animal research in the 1960s (Seligman and Maier, 1967). Dogs were subjected to inescapable electric shocks. When the barrier preventing their escape from these shocks was removed, the dogs continued to withstand them anyway and did not seek escape. Even if they accidentally avoided the shocks, they did not internalize this learning and continued to endure subsequent shocks. They had resigned themselves to their fate; they had 'learned helplessness'. The dogs, however, did 're-learn' how to escape after repeated 'teachings' by the researchers, in which the dogs were pushed, pulled or prodded away from the area being shocked. Martin Seligman has now coined another term, 'learned optimism', to encompass the dynamic of learning how to develop positive self-images (Seligman, 1990).

Michael Lerner (1986), a political scientist and psychotherapist, argues that a similar phenomenon occurs with persons living in risk conditions. He named this process 'surplus powerlessness', a surplus created by, but distinct from, external or objective conditions of powerlessness. An example of surplus powerlessness is provided in Box 2.3. Individuals internalize their objective or external powerlessness and create a potent psychological barrier to empowering action. They 'do not even engage in activities that meet their real needs. They begin to accept aspects of their world that are self-destructive to their own health and wellbeing, thinking that these are unalterable features of what they take to be "reality"' (Lerner, 1986). Part of this internalizing process is isolation, removing oneself from active group participation because of low self-esteem and high self-blame. Research affirms this process: poorer people internalize self-blame for their poverty, their self-esteem plummets and they isolate themselves from friends and colleagues (Auslander, 1988; Berkman, 1986; Cohen and Syme, 1985).

**Box 2.3:   Surplus powerlessness and women living
in inner-city housing**

Several years ago in a large inner-city housing estate, a community organizing
project had formed around food, gardens, housing and welfare. Many of the
women involved in this estate complained of having low self-esteem. A
principal reason for this was the fact that, by being on welfare, they had
ceased being autonomous, self-empowered individuals and had become a
form of public property. They had internalized their 'lesser eligibility', a key
concept in welfare policy that people on social assistance were only eligible for
income that was less than the lowest wage available in the job market. They
had become lesser persons. Not only did the women have low self-esteem;
they knew they had it, and they pinpointed one of the reasons for it: media
stereotypes about welfare recipients. These stereotypes came in two forms: on
Saturdays came the story of the super welfare heroine who transforms welfare
into a business and, by buying day-old bread and second-hand but functional
clothing, manages to virtually 'turn a profit'. On Wednesdays were the
'macaroni and cheese stories' about how horrible it was to barely subsist on
welfare. Just as society-at-large externalizes these stereotypes, many of the
women had internalized them. The result was 'surplus powerlessness', a
further dis-empowerment. With the first stereotype, they couldn't measure up
to the welfare heroine and so experienced themselves as personal failures.
With the second stereotype, their reality was consistently portrayed as bleak
and uncompromising. A key strategy in their empowerment was to reclaim,
and project publicly, positive images of their own lives and experiences. A key
role of the health promoter in this project was helping the women to gain the
resources, knowledge and access to networks that they needed to accomplish
this task. (Labonte, 1998)

There is increasing evidence that factors contributing to chronic anxiety
worsen health, especially in the context of grossly unequal societies. For
example, the rapid growth of income inequality in the UK from the 1970s
to the 1990s and the growth of social exclusion are directly implicated in
causing and sustaining health inequalities. Narrowing the gap in equali-
ties means taking action to address social exclusion using strategies that
use a range of social, economic and environmental interventions and the
empowerment of individuals and communities (Putnam et al., 1993;
Kawachi et al., 1997; Macleod et al., 1999).

Michael Lerner (1986) believed that specific group education could
overcome self-blame while improving health status and health behaviours. His research involved blue collar workers experiencing occupational stress. Compared to control groups, persons in the experimental
occupational 'stress groups' demonstrated statistically significant
improvements in such areas as social support, health behaviours, absen-
teeism and perceived power. The key construct, self-blame, decreased

significantly as social support behaviours among stress group participants improved. That 'stress groups' took place under union sponsorship may have been an important factor. Many stressors are embedded in the structure of work, and actions to remedy this problem requires an organized, political effort. Unions, through their collective bargaining, afford individual workers an opportunity to take collective actions on the 'structural' elements of work such as risk conditions, while the stress groups improved social support and coping behaviours. This raises the importance of creating effective political organizations to influence public and private policies that create the risk conditions in the first place.

Behavioural risk factors

People who live in risk conditions, and internalize this as psychosocial risk factors, are also more likely to have unhealthier lifestyles or behavioural risk factors, for example, smoking and consumption of high-fat foods which can serve as stress-coping 'rewards'. Indeed, Meredith Blaxter's UK research (1990) found that if people living in poor conditions did manage to change their health behaviours, but there was no change in their risk conditions, their self-reported health actually worsened! This shouldn't be taken to mean that we must end all forms of oppression before we can focus on the lifestyles of the oppressed. But it calls into question yet again the importance of how we conceptualize the relationship between individual behaviours and social conditions, and where we apportion the focus of our work as health promoters.

Finally, because people caught in this web of risk conditions and risk factors experience less social support and greater isolation, they are often less likely to be active in community groups or processes concerned with improving risk conditions in the first place (Auslander, 1988; Minkler, 1985). This 'feedback loop' reinforces isolation and self-blame, reinforcing the experience of disease or dis-ease. It is also one of the very reasons why an empowerment approach to health promotion has become both more popular and important in recent years. Such an approach, targeting people at greatest social disadvantage, seeks to engage these very people who, on their own, are the least likely to self-organize.

Implications to an empowering health promotion practice

Labonte (1998) identifies four important health promotion practice implications of the risk factors of health determinants, identified in Figure 2.1. First, at the level of national and international public policy, the question for health promotion is only partly one of how much wealth a nation creates. A nation needs sufficient national income or national resources to prevent physically compromising poverty. But once this is achieved, the more basic health promotion concern is how equitably that wealth and the decision-making power it provides is shared within the nation.

Second, working to overcome the learned helplessness or surplus powerlessness of less objectively powerful persons becomes important work, and in three senses:

- it is immediately healthful for the psychosocial wellbeing it creates;
- it is an essential first step in mobilizing community actions in support of those international and national policies that will create more economic and political fairness; and
- it may improve health behaviours over the longer term.

Third, there would be little disagreement among many health promoters that risk conditions are important, but there may be considerable disagreement over how they explain unequal health outcomes. While many health practitioners accept risk conditions as health determinants in their own right, others view them more as 'holding categories', statistically associated with increased rates of smoking, poor diet and indolence. These practitioners become interested in poverty, not for its own sake, but because poor people smoke more. As two researchers put it: that smoking rates are higher in lower-class persons should cause us to ask what is it about social class that causes smoking? (Evans and Stoddart, 1990). However, the really important question to ask, as far as health determinants are concerned, is 'What is it about political and economic practices that causes class?' For a focus on social class as holding categories for health behaviours fails to consider the enormity of health inequalities arising from poverty or social inequality, independent of health behaviour.

Fourth, accepting a social and environmental determinants agenda for health promotion does not mean that practitioners or the health sector have sole responsibility for action. Health professionals may begin their work with an individual or group around a physiological, behavioural or psychosocial risk factor, or around a risk condition. Health promoters must strip the pathways of health determinants back to their 'risk conditions' otherwise they will forever be treating the symptoms and never preventing the cause. The socio-environmental task is to locate these disease and behavioural risks in their psychosocial and socio-environmental contexts (for example, powerlessness, poverty and isolation), to recognize these contexts as independent health risks in their own right, and to recognize the importance of acting around all of the risk conditions. The key to addressing inequalities in health is in reducing the gap between rich and poor and in transforming unequal power relationships which are indicative of our society and working practices. Long term this requires political action on the causes of poverty such as unemployment through policies that influence, for example, welfare services, housing, transport and community health services. Whilst health promoters cannot be expected to change these long term goals by themselves, they do have a crucial role to play in the redistribution of power, the control over decisions and resources that influence people's lives and health. Short term, health promoters can reorientate their professional practice to enable individuals and communities to have greater influence over actions that can bring about social and political change. This is the process of community empowerment and is central to health promotion practice.

This chapter has outlined a simple interpretation of positive health and its implications for health promotion, described three different health promotion approaches, and explained a simple framework of risk conditions for health determinants, and what this means for an 'empowering' health promotion practice. To accept the challenges presented by the political health activist Rudolf Virchow, discussed in Chapter 1, these issues must be connected to how we as practitioners recognize and use power, and is the topic of Chapter 3. Then in Chapter 4 I take the discussion of power further to include the means to attaining power, empowerment, and situate these concepts within the context of health promotion practice.

3 Power Transformation and Health Promotion Practice

Empowerment is at the heart of the 'new' health promotion, and power is at the core of empowerment. Many health promoters have become more adept at understanding power relations in their work, but most still have a superficial understanding of the different meanings and practices of power. For health promotion practice to grow, we need to understand better how power suffuses the relationships between different stakeholders, and how programmes can transform unhealthy into healthy power relationships. In this book I use the term 'stakeholders' to mean people, groups and organizations who have some interest or influence in the programme. The primary stakeholders or beneficiaries are those people who are ultimately affected and at whom the programme is usually targeted, for example the community. The secondary stakeholders are the people or organizations that act as an intermediary in the delivery of the programme; they are the outside agents, for example health promoters.

To explain how power relationships can be transformed in a programme context I consider several different interpretations of social power: power-from-within (personal power as an inner strength or feeling of integrity); power-over (the ability to influence the actions of others, even against their will); and power-with (the ability to share forms of power-over to increase people's power-from-within). These interpretations allow further conclusions to be reached about community empowerment within a health promotion practice in Chapter 4.

What is power?

A common definition of power presents it as in the nature of power-over (people), 'the capacity of some persons to produce intended and foreseen effects on others' Wrong (1988: 2). This can exist in four different forms: authority, force, manipulation and persuasion. The German social scientist, Max Weber (1947: 152), offers a similar definition of power as 'the probability that one actor within a social relationship will be in a position to carry out his own will despite resistance.' Weber identifies two forms of power that he also closely links to conflict; one where conflict is absent, the other where the resistance of others must be overcome. The anthropologist,

Richard Adams (1977: 387), extends the idea of power further by vesting it in both individuals and social groups, as '… the ability of a person or social unit to influence the conduct and decision-making of another through the control over energetic forms in the latter's environment …'. These interpretations are all variations on how power is commonly referenced in the social science literature: one person having influence and mastery over another.

To exercise choice is the simplest form of power. This may involve the trivial choices of everyday life or the more critical choices and decisions which influence health. To the extent that our personal choices constrain those of others, it becomes an exercise of power-over. People with the ability to control decisions at the macro (political and economic) level, for example, condition and constrain the ability of people to exercise control or choice at the micro (individual and group) levels. Sometimes we willingly accord people this macro-level ability, as in legislation to prevent or punish crimes against people.

Zero-sum and non-zero-sum forms of power

The type of power I have so far discussed is based on viewing it as a finite entity. Zero-sum power exists when one can only possess x amount of power to the extent that someone else has the absence of an equivalent amount. It is therefore a 'win/lose' situation. My power-over you, plus your absence of that power, equals zero (thus the term 'zero-sum'). I win and you lose. For you to gain power, you must seize it from me. If you can, you win and I lose. This concept of power, in which leverage is used to raise the position of one person or group while simultaneously lowering it for another person or group, is particularly dominant in western thinking.

Zero-sum power is often used in association with economic or political accounts where power is equated to wealth and income and subsequently authority and status. At any one time there will be only so much wealth possessed within a society. This distribution and the decision-making authority that goes with it is zero-sum. One has authority or social status by virtue of others not having it. There is a degree of flexibility here, however, since someone may have authority or status in one situation, relative to others, but not in another. At the same time there are dominant social forms of status or privilege, such as class, gender, education, ethnic background, age and even physical ability or sexual preference, which tend to structure power-over relations in most social situations.

The role of health promotion in this zero-sum construction of power is to assist groups to gain power, meaning here more control over resources or decision-making that influence their health, from other groups. Within communities, this can become a difficult issue. David Zakus and Catherine Lysack (1998), two Canadian health researchers, argue that health promotion practice that works from a zero-sum construction of power increases 'unhealthy' competition between people and groups and decreases 'healthy' community cohesion. They suggest that 'community empowerment' is a contradiction in terms and that by empowering some at the expense of others, health promoters are actually breaking down the ties that hold a community together.

In Chapter 4 I argue that 'community' is not homogeneous but by its very nature consists of competing heterogeneous individuals and groups, and that health promoters cannot avoid their work empowering some whilst not others. The point raised by Zakus and Lysack, however, highlights the ethical and political dilemma of which groups, at the expense of others, should get priority of the limited resources and assistance from the health promoters. This problem is confounded if the group is unpopular or involved in illegal or unpalatable activities such as drug use or child abuse. The role of the health promoter is to be non-judgemental and self-reflecting in their work. Recalling the previous chapter's discussion of social justice in Box 2.2, priority needs to go to those groups facing the greatest inequalities in health outcomes and socio-economic opportunities.

There is another important concept of power, however, one that regards it not as fixed and finite, but as infinite and expanding. These 'non-zero-sum' forms of power are 'win/win', since they are based on the idea that if any one person or group gains, everyone else gains also. Knowledge, trust, caring and other aspects of our social relationships with one another are examples of non-zero-sum power.

Perhaps unsurprisingly, health promoters often gravitate towards the non-zero-sum formulation. Certainly, much of the recent discourse of health promotion, by emphasizing '… participation, caring, sharing and responsibility to others', addresses the exercise of power in which all people can benefit. Power is no longer seen as a finite commodity, such as wealth, or as the comparative status and authority that this might confer. Rather this non-zero-sum power takes the form of relationship behaviours based on respect, generosity, service to others, a free flow of information and the commitment to the ethics of caring and justice. The role of the health promoter in this construction of power is to use these attributes to engender them in others and to transfer power between groups by encouraging individuals to access information by themselves, in part by providing better access to resources and information, for example, through an Internet link.

Health promotion practice simultaneously involves zero-sum and non-zero-sum formulations of power. Power cannot be given but communities can be enabled by health promoters to gain or seize power from others. To do this, the role of health promoters is to first identify their own power base (access to resources and influence) and to understand how this can be appropriately acted upon to enable others to gain power through their own endeavours. It is the relationship between the stakeholders that is empowering and leads to the 'community' developing the ability and opportunities to seize control over the influences on their lives and health.

I will explore further below how both of these forms of power are present in health promotion programmes and the transformative ways in which they can be used to empower others.

Three faces of power

To better understand how social power is exercised in both a positive manner (the sharing of control with others) and a negative manner (the use of control to exert influence over others), it is helpful to reconsider zero-sum and non-zero-sum power. Zero-sum power should be viewed as power-over and non-zero-sum as power-from-within and power with. Power with is really the transformative use of power-over. This is complex, so consider first how philosopher Thomas Wartenberg (1990) describes the two-faced nature of power: power-to, or our abilities to do or accomplish something by ourselves; and power-over, or the ability to affect the actions or ideas of others despite their resistance. Starhawk (1990) takes the concept of power-to and further subdivides it in two: power-from-within, or one's personal power, an inner energy that might include self-knowledge, self-discipline and self-esteem; and power-with, in which power-over transformatively increases other people's power-from-within, rather than to dominate or exploit them. I illustrate this in the story in Box 3.2 (see page 41) of the community nurse who used her professional power-over to gently persuade women in a rooming house to develop more of their own capacities (strengthening their power-from-within) so that they could become their own advocates.

Power-from-within

Power-from-within can be described as an experience of 'self', a personal power or some inner sense of integrity or 'truth' (Labonte, 1996). An example of this form of power is provided in Box 3.1. Others argue that power-from-within is gained from philosophical, religious and spiritual sources (Morriss, 1987; Wartenberg, 1990). Power-from-within is also known as individual, personal or psychological empowerment and many definitions of this concept have been developed in the field of community psychology in westernized countries. Generally, these describe power-from-within, or personal empowerment, as gaining (a sense of) control over one's life (Rissel, 1994). Recall in Box 2.1 (see page 17) that experiencing this sense of control is how many people, from a variety of cultures, partly describe how they experience 'being healthy'. Starhawk's description of power-from-within is similar; she likens it to '... our sense of mastery we develop as young children ...', but also to something deeper '... our sense of bonding with other human beings, and with the environment' (1990: 10). The goal of psychological empowerment is to increase feelings of value and a sense of mastery. The individualization of this concept can lead to approaches that aim to increase the notion of 'self', ignoring how power-over can constrain experiences of marginalized groups. Power-from-within is not concerned with access to or control over resources. Individuals can therefore become more powerful from within and do not necessarily have to accumulate power as money, or status or authority.

***

Box 3.1: Power-from-within in Maori people

Maori people in Aotearoa, New Zealand suffer in the same ways that other indigenous colonized people suffer. Many of them are poor, unemployed, victimized and self-victimizing with alcoholism and abuse. Sympathetic Pakeha (as Maori refer to others) go to great lengths to decry the powerlessness and impoverishment that create their poor health. They want to focus attention on what we now call the 'determinants of health', poverty, pollution, discrimination, all of which are effects of a social system whose dominant paradigm is power-over. Pakeha health workers do not want to blame poor Maori heath on their high smoking rates, poor nutrition habits, bad-parenting skills or lack of family planning. But to many Maori, this explanation is little better than the lifestyle victim-blaming it replaces. While they lack the legislative authority to reorganize their communities as autonomous political systems, many Maori are doing so anyway. In one instance, they used government funds for a computer training programme for unemployed youth to develop their own census of every Maori woman, man and child. Their intention is to keep tabs on the individuals in their communities. When a person begins to run into difficulties, counsellors and healers from their extended families can act to re-integrate them in ways that are more in keeping with Maori culture. The Maori leaders who developed this programme were asked: 'How can you do this? Only elected governments can create such a census. You don't have the authority or power to do this.' They replied, 'We act as if we have the authority and the power. And in acting this way, we develop the very authority and power you say we do not possess.' There is even a name for this stance: tino rangitiratanga, or 'acting from the position of Maori chieftaincy,' more commonly defined as Maori self-determination, or what we would call power-from-within. (Labonte, 1998)

Power-over

Power-over describes social relationships in which one party is made to do what another party wishes them to, despite their resistance and even if it may not be in their best interests. Starhawk describes power-over in its clearest form as '… the power of the prison guard, of the gun, power that is ultimately backed by force' (1990: 9). The exercise of power-over does not always have to be negative. State legislation to control the spread of diseases, to impose fines for unhealthy behaviour such as smoking in a public place, or even to redistribute market income to prevent poverty, are all examples of what we consider 'healthy' power-over. At issue is, whose choices are constrained and why? There is no easy answer to this question. This is something health promoters need to deliberate for themselves in light of the following questions: Does this power-over constrain/improve the health and wellbeing of society's poorest or most marginalized groups? Does this power-over constrain/make the distribution of decision-making authority more equitable in the community or society?

Power-over can take different forms depending on how it is used to exert control or to influence others. Many writers settle on three function-ally distinct operations of power-over: dominance, or the direct power to control people's choices, usually by force or its threat; exploitation, or the indirect power to control people's choices through economic relations, in which those who control capital (primarily money) also have control over those who do not; and hegemony, or the ability of a dominant group to control the actions and behaviours of others by intense persuasion.

Hegemonic power is that form of power-over that is invisible and inter-nalized such that it is structured into our everyday lives and taken for granted (Foucault, 1979). To Foucault, a prominent theorist and commen-tator on power, the only form of resistance to hegemonic power was a concealment of one's life from those in authority. For example, the hidden actions of a prisoner from his gaolers or a single mother living in poor housing hiding a messy room or her sick child from a health visitor (Bloor and McIntosh, 1990). Persons living in conditions of hegemonic power-over, of oppression and exploitation, internalize these conditions as being their personal responsibility. This internalization increases their own self-blame and decreases their self-esteem. This internalization can lead to false consciousness, a failing to utilize the power one has and failing to acquire powers that one can acquire (Morriss, 1987). Hegemonic power-over is inherently unhealthy, because it shuts down critical thinking, public debate and the possibility of change. One of the subtle ways in which health promoters participate in hegemonic power-over is when they continually impose their ideas of what are important health prob-lems without listening to what community members think are important health concerns. For example, people come to think about health as 'dis-ease' or 'lifestyles' and only begin to expand their ideas about health when they are carefully asked: what does it really mean for you?

In a programme context there are two other forms of power-over that are discussed:

- coercion is an overt and explicit form when a dominant group (an out-side agent) maintains its power-over by forcing people to do things against their will; and

- consent when a dominant group maintains power-over by gaining the consent of subordinate groups or individuals. It does this by distorting, concealing or deflecting a real understanding of the power relation and the way in which it works. This can occur in partnerships where one group has dominance, takes a paternalistic approach or lacks respect for the other partner; discussed further in Chapter 7 (Jones and Sidell, 1997: 51).

Power-with

Power-with describes a different set of social relationships, in which power-over is used carefully and deliberately to increase other people's power-from-within, rather than to dominate or exploit them. Thomas Wartenberg (1990) provides the example of the relationship between parent and child as an exemplar of the transformative use of power-over. Power-over transforms to power-with only when it has effectively reached its end, when the submissive person in the relationship has accrued enough power-from-within to exercise his or her own choices and decisions. Western feminist theory also supports the concept of power-with in that the greater the development of each individual the more able, effective and less dependent on others they become (Katz, 1984; Swift and Levin, 1987). Wartenberg (1990) argues that feminist theory holds that even in the most male-dominated, power-over society, women have power, the power-from-within. Feminist theory claims that although women are not socially dominant, they do have special skills and inner strengths that have enabled them to act in invaluable ways. Once one has accepted this, Wartenberg's (1990: 188) argument that '... the seemingly contradictory claim that women both have and lack power-over in a male dominated society...' can be seen to contain an important insight into the role of women. Power-over becomes a decentred notion: a person may hold a great deal of authority in one aspect of their life but possess very little in other aspects of their life.

Starhawk identifies the source of power-with as '... the willingness of others to listen to our ideas' (1990: 10). The person with the power-over chooses not to command or exert control, but to suggest and to begin a discussion that will increase the other's sense of power-from-within. The parent offers advice, guides and helps the child to develop its own power-from-within, its abilities and inner strengths. It is patronizing to equate health promoters' relationship to communities as parent/child. Yet, with respect to some facets of community members' lives, health promoters may have knowledge and resources useful to them and may give priority to communities that are relatively powerless. Rather than a simple transfer of resources and information, then, health promoters' relationship with community members should involve an offering of advice and strategies to develop both the psychological empowerment (self-esteem and self-confidence) of individuals and the collective empowerment of the group. The transformative use of power-over demands a great deal of self-vigilance and self-discipline by all persons in the relationship, but in particular by the initially more dominant person. Otherwise the relationship can remain as power-over, for example, legitimate or expert power that does not acknowledge that others in the relationship may have their own expertise can lead to a patronizing inducement of dependency. Linden (1994) suggests that the doctor and patient relationship is unequal where all competence is considered to belong to one party and that this is often between a male 'expert' and a female 'target' or patient. Thus the woman voluntarily surrenders to the unspoken claim of medical (expert) power. The doctor has a monopoly of knowledge even though that knowledge concerns the patient's own body. Medicalization works within the frame of this double power relation, differences of knowledge and gender. The attributes of health are viewed as an individual 'case' and the diagnosis is made on that basis. Thus the medical model serves to protect the legitimate and expert power of the professional.

Ann Robertson and Meredith Minkler (1994) describe the professional empowering relationship as one of facilitating communities and individuals to identify their health requirements, solutions and action to these solutions. In practice this role is the transformation of power-over to power-with which requires, in part, a non-coercive dialogue in the identification and resolution of problems and the use of the health promoter's power-over to strengthen community and individual autonomy. An example of this is provided in Box 3.2.

Powerlessness

I cannot conclude this discussion without mentioning powerlessness, or the absence of power, whether imagined or real. Powerlessness can be an individual concept with the expectancy that the behaviour of a person cannot determine the outcomes they seek. Powerlessness is viewed as a continuous interaction between the person and his or her environment. It combines an attitude of self-blame, a sense of generalized distrust, a feeling of alienation from resources for social influence, an experience of disenfranchisement and economic vulnerability, and a sense of hopelessness in socio-political struggle (Kieffer, 1984). Powerlessness may also be viewed as a result of the passive acceptance of oppressive cultural 'givens', or the surrender to a 'culture of silence' (Freire, 1973). Paulo Freire believed that the individual becomes powerless in assuming the role of 'object' acted upon by the environment, rather the 'subject' acting in and on the world. As such, the individual alienates himself or herself from participation in the construction of social reality (Wallerstein, 1992).

> ### Box 3.2: Power transformation through health promotion practice
>
> Female residents of a rooming house in Toronto, Canada, complained of men demanding sexual favours in exchange for letting them gain access to the bathroom. The women requested assistance from the community nurse to use her authority and professional status to lend credibility to their complaints. The nurse agreed. She also advised the women that, after her initial assistance, they would have to pursue the issue with the appropriate authorities themselves, and she would mentor them to do so. In this way the nurse strengthened the power-from-within of the community (the women), first by using her power-over (status, authority) and then by supporting them to act as their own advocates. But in laying down her power-over condition ('I'll do this, but only if you'll learn how to do it yourselves … ') she exercised her power with the intent of increasing the power-from-within of the others (the women) in the relationship. This is the hallmark of the transformative use of power, the intent with which it is exercised. (Labonte, 1998).

The powerless often experience little leverage on the events and conditions that impinge on their existence, either directly or through access to resources that guarantee survival, decrease discomfort, and enable change and betterment in one's life (Kroeker, 1995). Kieffer provides an expression of the daily experience of individual powerlessness by Sharon, a Native American living in Harlem: 'It would never have occurred to me to have expressed an opinion on anything … It was inconceivable that my opinion had any value … that's lower than powerlessness … You don't even know the word "power" exists'(1984: 16).

The health promoter's first challenge in these situations is to strengthen individuals' power-from-within, partly by identifying their own sources of power-over. People's power or powerlessness, for example, is always 'relative' to others in their community or country. People may hold a great deal of authority in one aspect of their life but possess very little in other aspects. An immigrant man may hold the position of a community leader or hereditary chief within his own community, but within his workplace have only a low-paying menial job with little responsibility or status. In the same way, the stakeholders of a programme may bring with them a great deal of power in the form of authority and control within their community. These individuals can be an important factor in enabling others to take control of the influences on their lives and health. An example of this is the use of local leaders to manage programmes assisted by 'technical experts' to improve the skills and competencies of these individuals. I discuss the issue of local leadership in a health promotion programme context in Chapter 7.

Rather than begin their work from the perspective that people who are, in general terms, 'relatively' economically and politically powerless, health promoters need to look for, and work from, areas in people's lives in which they are 'relatively' powerful. The health promoter's second challenge is to assist individuals to organize collectively to increase their collective exercise of power-over.

In this chapter I have explored some of power's different meanings, and shown how they pertain to health promotion practice. In the next chapter I discuss the second theme of this book, community empowerment, and show how this concept can be used to support an empowering health promotion practice.

4 Community Empowerment and Health Promotion Practice

In this chapter I discuss the concept of community empowerment and how it can be successfully applied to health promotion practice to provide a more empowering approach. In fact, community empowerment is two concepts: community and empowerment. Before I discuss empowerment, I will first define what is considered to be a 'community'.

The concept of community

Community has many contradictory definitions. An analysis of these by Bell and Newby (1978) concludes that, although there is a lack of agreement beyond the idea of community involving people, the majority of definitions do include the following components: area, common ties and social interaction. The discussion by Bell and Newby (1978) goes beyond the customary view of community as a place where people live such as a village, neighbourhood or town because such areas can be just an aggregate of non-connected people.

It is important to recognize that the precise meaning of community will likely vary from area to area and from individual to individual. Two different writers, Jayakumar Christian (1993) and Stephen Githumbi (1993), illustrate the fundamental importance of social relations in two very different cultural contexts. Christian states that within an Asian Indian context people '... define themselves by the community ... to which they belong' (1993: 6). Likewise, Githumbi states that within an African context most people associate their '... identity and wellbeing ... on how much a person is 'in tune' with their community' (1993: 6). Githumbi quotes an African saying that captures the notion of community: 'I am because you are; if you are not, then I cannot be'.

The main issue for health promoters undertaking community empowerment is whether the community is a social, geographic or demographic concept. Although a community can possess all of these elements, writers such as Bell and Newby (1978) argue the emphasis should be placed on the changing and dynamic nature of social relations. Barbara Israel and her colleagues, who have done extensive research on community empowerment in the US (1994), characterize a community locale as possessing the following elements: membership, common symbol systems, shared values and norms, mutual influence, shared needs, and shared emotional connection. The element of 'shared needs' is especially important to the subject of this book, as I interpret empowerment as a continuum based on a community's shared needs later in this chapter.

Penelope Hawe (1994), based on her community health research, argues that rather than relying on what health promoters write about 'community', we should interpret how they have used the concept; for example, the way in which they evaluate their programmes. She suggests that three distinct approaches to community can be observed. The first is community interpreted as a population, for example, women, men and youth (demographic). The second is community interpreted as a setting, for example, schools, hospitals and workplaces (geographic). She describes the third approach as the '... capacity to work towards solutions to its own community-identified problems ...' (Hawe, 1994: 201). The first two interpretations represent populations and settings approaches commonly used in top-down health promotion programming. The third interpretation is more commonly associated with bottom-up, community development or community empowerment programmes and defines community less by place or setting and more by social interaction, common ends and needs.

This interpretation of community is further supported by Jim Ward, an organizer with experience with 'street communities' in Brisbane, Sydney and Toronto. He describes this third aspect of communities as 'A group of people perceiving common needs and problems, that acquires a sense of identity focused around these problems and that a common set of objectives grow out of these identified issues' (Ward, 1987: 18).

What can be concluded from this is that geographic communities consist of heterogeneous individuals who may organize into specific groups to take collective action towards shared and specific goals. The diversity of individuals and groups within a geographic community can create problems in regard to the selection of representation by its members (Zakus and Lysack, 1998). Health promoters need to carefully consider who are 'legitimate' representatives of a community. Those individuals who have the energy, time and motivation to become involved in programme activities may, in fact, not be supported by other community members and may be considered as self-interested élites. The dominant minority may dictate the community needs unless adequate precautions are taken to involve marginalized populations. Zakus and Lysack (1998) also point out that some groups may prefer to remain anonymous as they are accustomed to being ignored or are unaware of the opportunities offered by a programme. It is a paradox of empowerment approaches that the most marginalized populations are often unable to articulate their needs or are unaware of opportunities and, as a result, often become excluded from the benefits and opportunities that health promotion programmes can represent.

The importance of recognizing that community members can be heterogeneous and yet still have the ability to share needs and interests is reflected in the difficulties experienced within aboriginal health services in Australia. Aboriginal communities are often a collection of families, language groups or clans who can be in competition and who may be geographically isolated. The term 'community' was applied to such settlements by bureaucratic intellectuals because it provided a convenient label for the assimilation of different concepts and for a heterogeneous group of people (Scrimgeour, 1997). The assumption that different aboriginal groups were homogeneous led to a lack of cooperation, direction and collective action between its members. The definition of 'community' was based on administrative convenience rather than traditional structures and this created an atmosphere in which empowerment was more difficult to achieve.

Heterogeneous groups can actually become more of a community through the process of programme planning, to the extent that programme aims and objectives reflect, at least in part, shared interests and needs of members in a given locality. These become the shared focus for community action. Individual, family or clan-based differences may then be set aside as programme participants begin to create a shared identity around the more tightly focused programme aims. Involving programme participants in the identification of issues and concerns is therefore crucial to ensure that the programme aims and objectives are relevant and capable of overcoming any divisions that might exist between participants. This does not preclude problems of conflict arising during programme planning and implementation, an issue taken up later, but can help to reduce it. The members of the newly formed community organize and mobilize themselves around the programme which, in turn, facilitates the means by which they empower themselves. This is enhanced when communities have shared needs, social networks and the desire to gain power. If these elements do not exist, health promoters need to strengthen social relationships and organizations that might assist the community to identify its own needs and problems.

I have so far argued that the concept of 'community' includes several key characteristics and have summarized these points in Box 4.1. In this book I use a definition of community as existing in organized groups that are important enough to their individual members that they identify themselves, in part, by their group membership. This interpretation implies that within the geographic or spatial dimensions of community, multiple communities exist and each individual may belong to several different communities at the same time.

Heterogeneous individuals are able to achieve collective action through a process that involves personal action and the development of small groups, organizations and networks, in effect the development of community as discussed above. For a group of disparate individuals to gain power through this process its members must be able to put aside their differences and focus on their shared interests and concerns. When this process leads to achieving social and political change it is most often described as the continuum of community empowerment, and it is this that I explore next in relation to health promotion practice.

Box 4.1:   The key characteristics of 'community'

- A spatial dimension, that is, a place or locale.
- Non-spatial dimensions (interests, issues, identities) that involve people who otherwise make up heterogeneous and disparate groups.
- Social interactions that are dynamic and bind people into relationships with one another.
- Identification of shared needs and concerns that can be achieved through a process of collective action.

Three levels of empowerment

Empowerment in the broadest sense is '… the process by which disadvantaged people work together to increase control over events that determine their lives' (Werner, 1988). Most definitions of empowerment give the term a similarly positive value, and have been largely developed by psychologists in industrialized countries in the areas of neighbourhood empowerment and community mental health (Torre, 1986; Rappaport, 1987; Swift and Levin, 1987). These definitions embody the notion that empowerment must come from within a group and cannot be given to a group or community.

The over-use and misuse of the term 'empowerment' has led to it having a lesser significance and a diminished meaning in recent years. To provide clarity to this concept it is useful to consider the different levels of empowerment suggested by several theorists (for example, Rissel, 1994; Israel et al., 1994). Christopher Rissel includes a heightened or increased level of psychological empowerment as a part of community empowerment. He also argues that community empowerment includes '… a political action component in which members have actively participated, and the achievement of some redistribution of resources or decision making favourable to the community or group in question' (Rissel, 1994). Barbara Israel and her colleagues (1994) similarly identify psychological and political action as two levels of community empowerment, but include a third and intermediary level between them, that of organizational empowerment. Their analysis of this level draws heavily from democratic management theory. An empowered organization is one that is democratically managed, its members share information and control over decisions and are involved in the design, implementation and control of efforts toward goals defined by group consensus. It is an essential link between empowered individuals and effective political action.

Community empowerment thus includes personal (psychological) empowerment, organizational empowerment and broader social and political changes. Nina Wallerstein (1992), one of the more influential American writers on health and empowerment, further views this concept as a synergistic interaction between all three of these levels. Community empowerment is both an individual and a group phenomena. It is also a dynamic process that never ends, involving continual shifts in personal empowerment (power-from-within) and changes in power-over relations between different social groups and decision-makers in the broader society.

Community empowerment as an outcome can vary, for example, as a redistribution of resources (Rappaport, 1984; Rody, 1988; Oakley, 1991), a decrease in individuals' or groups' powerlessness (Kieffer, 1984; Rappaport, 1985) or success in achieving a programme's goals (Plough and Olafson, 1994; Purdey et al., 1994; Rudner-Lugo, 1996). But it is as a process that it is most consistently viewed in the literature, for example, '… a social-action process that promotes participation of people, organizations and communities towards the goals of increased individual and community control, political efficacy, improved quality of life and social justice' (Wallerstein, 1992). As a process, community empowerment is best considered as a continuum representing progressively more organized and broadly-based forms of social and collective action, and it is to the continuum model of empowerment that I now turn.

Community empowerment as a five-point continuum

Community empowerment has been most consistently viewed in the health promotion literature as a five-point continuum model comprising the following elements:

1 Personal action.
2 The development of small mutual groups.
3 Community organizations.
4 Partnerships.
5 Social and political action. (Jackson et al., 1989; Labonte, 1990).

The continuum model offers a simple, linear interpretation of what is a dynamic and complex concept and articulates the various levels of empowerment from personal, to organizational through collective (community) action. Each point on the continuum can be viewed as an outcome in itself, as well as a progression onto the next point. If not achieved the outcome is stasis or even a move back to the preceding point on the continuum. In particular, the establishment of community organizations is a crucial step in the process of community empowerment and it is at

Figure 4.1 Community empowerment as a continuum

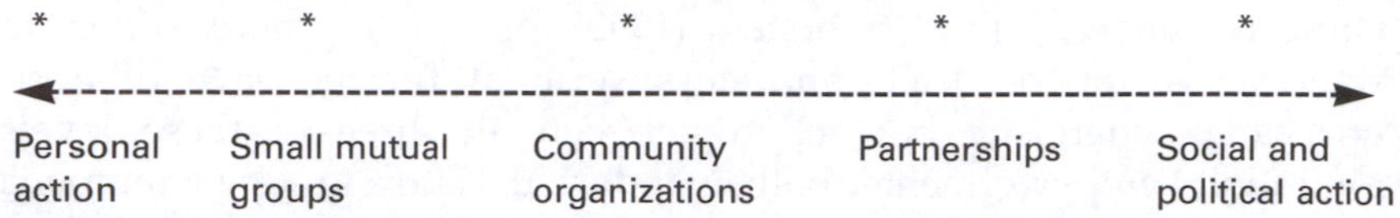

```
   *             *              *              *              *

◄----------------------------------------------------------------------►

Personal      Small mutual    Community      Partnerships   Social and
action        groups          organizations                 political action
```

Source: Laverack, 1999: 92.

this point that individuals can develop the necessary skills in resource mobilization, leadership, problem assessment and critical awareness.

The continuum model has remained unchallenged in the literature, although different authors have used slightly different terminology which essentially hold the same meaning (Labonte, 1998; Rissel, 1994), and has been used by health promotion practitioners to explain how community empowerment can potentially be maximized as people progress from individual to collective action. I blend the previous interpretations of the community empowerment continuum and provide an adapted version that is relevant to the subject of this book in Figure 4.1.

I will now briefly discuss how health promoters can use this model to build more empowered communities at each point on the continuum.

1 Empowering individuals for personal action

The process of community empowerment can begin at any point along the continuum, but for persons experiencing a high degree of 'relative powerlessness' it often starts with a personal action that builds a greater sense of power-from-within. Only by participating in small groups or organizations can individual community members better define, analyse and act on issues of concern. In everyday life a personal action and subsequent participation in the continuum can begin through a triggered response to an emotional or symbolic experience in a person's life, such as the siting of an industrial facility (Kieffer, 1984). In health promotion programmes the basis for personal action and participation is often developed during the planning phase through an identification of participants' own needs and problems, and later developed as aims and objectives. It is important that programmes use approaches to build in a structure as well as a personal way forward towards collective action and organization. If practitioners only focus on the individual they risk making the issue personal and if they only focus on the structural issues they run the risk of neglecting the immediate needs of many people.

Programmes that do not address community concerns and that do not involve the community in the process of problem assessment and decision-making, particularly in marginalized communities, have been shown not to achieve their purpose (Rifkin, 1990).

2 Empowering individuals for the development of small mutual groups

The development of small mutual groups by concerned individuals is the start of collective action. This provides an opportunity for the health promoter to assist the individual to gain skills and is a locus for developing stronger social support systems and opportunity networks, interpersonal connectedness and social cohesion (Putnam et al., 1993). An example of this situation, taken from North America, is provided in Box 4.2.

Box 4.2:   Organizing East African women on the issue of female genital mutilation

In recent years, large communities of refugees from East Africa have settled in several European and North American cities. Among some of these refugee communities the practice of female genital mutilation (FGM) is still common. On one hand, opposition to this practice could be seen as a dominant culture imposing its own standards. On the other hand, FGM has also been decried by African women and men on grounds of gender oppression. A mental health worker found herself straddling this political tightrope. She offered one-to-one counselling services through the auspices of an agency dealing with victims of torture. Concerns about FGM arose during some of the counselling sessions. The worker organized support groups for these women, which gradually increased their outward-looking orientation, including advocacy work on the issue of FGM. She also organized an interagency group of health and government organizations that could assist in the lobbying efforts of the women themselves. Direct community organizing around FGM was taken on by a women's health centre with a strong commitment to ethno-racial minorities. As the advocacy and organizing initiatives grew more complex, a multicultural health consultant with the local Council, with more experience in advocacy, became involved. She worked with other organizations to advance arguments to include FGM within the Criminal Code, and to treat its practice as an instance of child abuse. (Labonte, 1998)

The role of the practitioner at this point of the continuum is to bring people together in small groups around issues which they feel are important to their lives, in a manner that is not too controlling. These include:

• Self-help groups organized around a specific problem such as bereavement support groups and Alcoholics Anonymous. Members usually have a shared knowledge and interest in the problem, are participatory and supportive and the groups are often set-up and managed by the participants.

- Community health groups which usually come together to campaign on a specific issue such as environmental pollution, dog fouling in the community, or transport needs of socially excluded groups such as the aged. People are motivated to come together either for reactive or proactive reasons, usually for short-term periods. However these groups can also form long-lasting associations such as NIMBYs (Not In My Back Yard) in regard to issues like the siting of waste dumps.
- Community development health projects such as neighbourhood-based projects set up to address issues of local concern, such as poor housing, and with an appointed and paid community health worker (discussed further in Jones and Sidell, 1997: 29).

This is a complex and slow process that requires a sense of trust between the different members, and it may take many years before individuals feel comfortable in a group environment.

It is through the support of small groups that many people find a 'voice' and are able to participate in a more formal way to achieve the goals of social and political change. However, the membership of small groups is not homogeneous and conflict regarding internal issues does arise, especially during the shift from an inward (self-help) to an outward (social action) orientation.

Ronald Labonte (1998) provides an example of this in a community garden project in Toronto, Canada, which involved single mothers on social assistance. The group conflict was based on the importance of the garden. Some of the mothers saw the garden as a meeting place where they organized themselves to eventually become strong enough to address broader issues of social change influencing their lives. Other mothers saw the garden for the simple purpose of growing vegetables. Both activities, the self-help garden and the social mobilization it could create, are important empowerment outcomes. This example raises the important issue of how small groups can become focused on individual problems and not the deeper socio-environmental causes of poverty and powerlessness.

Problem assessment builds capacity when the identification of problems, solutions to the problems and actions to resolve the problems are carried out by the community. When these skills do not exist or are weak, the role of the practitioner will be to assist the community to make an assessment of its own problems. A number of participatory methodologies have evolved specifically for this purpose, including Rapid Rural Appraisal, Participatory Rural Appraisal and other assessment procedures (Marsden et al., 1994).

Health promoters must be prepared to listen to what the community wants; they may not necessarily like what they hear, but they must be committed to moving forward and building upon these issues.

3 Empowering groups for the development of community organizations

Community organization structures include small groups such as church and youth groups, community councils, united peasant farms and farmers' cooperatives, water users' and drinking water associations. These are the organizational elements in which people come together in order to socialize and to address their concerns. Community organizations are not only larger than small mutual groups, they also have an established structure, more functional leadership and the ability to organize their members to mobilize resources. Community organizations are crucial to the continuum because at this point individuals have the opportunity to gain the skills and networks necessary to allow small groups to make the transition to partnerships and later to social and political action.

While small groups generally focus inwards on the needs of its immediate members, community organizations focus outwards to the broader environment that creates those needs in the first place, or offers the means (resources, opportunities) to resolving them. Individuals become more critically aware of the broader issues in addition to learning the skills for assessing their immediate problems and needs. Many strategies that have become established for practitioners to develop skills in raising awareness about the broader social and political issues that influence the lives of individuals are based on the work of educationalist Paulo Freire. It is a process of emancipation through learning or education and has been adopted as an approach in many programmes including health education (Werner, 1988) and community development (Hope and Timmel, 1988).

Community organizations also enable people to progress along the empowerment continuum by improving the ability of small groups to raise resources. In Box 4.3 I provide an established example of the Seniors' Mobilization Project in North America that used community organizations to gain access to resources. It is worthwhile revisiting this example because it illustrates the role of the practitioner as a link between resources and the community, assisting the community members to 'map' or identify their internal resources (skills, knowledge and different forms of power) to help them build from a position of strength.

Box 4.3: The Seniors' Mobilization Project

A seniors' community outreach worker was hired by a community health centre. She began the housing project by conducting a community survey of seniors, announcing the door-to-door survey through a mail-out to all seniors in the area and posters in their buildings. The mail-out and posters included pictures of the worker, so people would not be fearful of opening their doors to a 'stranger'. The survey was structured, and solicited seniors' ideas about what could be done to make their lives and their living situation healthier, and which of the suggestions, created from an earlier survey, they would like to focus and work on.

On this basis the Seniors' Mobilization Project petitioned the government postal service to return the mailbox that had been removed from their buildings (it had been replaced with a post box stand well away from where most seniors resided). Seniors also initiated a low cost taxi service and part-time use of a vehicle belonging to a social service organization to assist them in leaving the housing project to go to nearby stores for shopping. Recreational services were minimal and the seniors organized their own committee to provide regular weekly activities. The seniors' group also initiated a neighbourhood recycling programme, created an advocacy anti-poverty group, and improved landscaping by the building managers. The organizer, and project members, reported that the organizing effort succeeded in mobilizing many participants because it worked on clear and short-term goals identified by residents, and supported issue oriented committees on such larger problem areas such as hunger, poverty and poor transportation only after initial 'successes' were experienced. The reasoning behind this stratagem is that initial short-term successes are needed to mobilize a previously unorganized group. Related to this belief, initial meetings on ideas defined by the survey did not require any ongoing commitment on the part of those who attended. Requiring commitment too early in the process could have scared many people away. (NYCHPRU, 1993)

The development of community organizations and local leadership are also closely connected and both play an important role in the development of small mutual groups and community organizations. The problem of selecting appropriate leadership is discussed by Goodman et al. (1998), who argue that a pluralistic approach in the community – one where there is an interplay between the positional leaders, those who have been elected or appointed and the reputational leaders, those who informally serve the community – has a better chance of leading to community capacity. However, this situation can create conflict; for example, in Fiji, I found that people were willing to openly identify that traditional (positional) leadership was weak and that this was mainly due to poor capacity, support and communication between the leaders, the community and organizations outside the community. However, through discussion the community was able to identify a number of realistic solutions to these weaknesses, for example leadership training, and to address the issue of conflict resolution between clan leaders (Laverack, 2003).

4 Empowering community organizations to develop partnerships

To be effective in influencing 'higher level' policy decision-making, community organizations need to link with other groups sharing similar concerns. Community organizations, by forming partnerships, can strengthen social networks, better compete for limited resources and increase support and participation in the concerns of other member organizations. The purpose of partnerships are to allow community organizations to grow beyond their own local concerns and to take a stronger position on broader issues through networking and advocacy.

The key empowerment issue is to remain focused on the shared concern that brings the groups together, and not on the individual needs or issues of the different groups in the partnership. The example of a partnership that floundered for lack of clarity on this important point is illustrated by a practitioner who, in a large city in Canada, convened a committee on housing and health with activists from housing rights groups. These groups wanted safer, better heated and ventilated, more affordable housing. The practitioner desired her agency to be more relevant to the issues expressed by these community groups. The housing and health partnership committee met for a year, documenting with studies and literature reviews that the activists' concerns were legitimate. The report then went through a prolonged process of internal review by her organization management. Eventually, the recommendations were rewritten, and watered down in a completely non-challenging, non-committal way. By this time the community groups had withdrawn from the partnership, feeling that their demands had not been honoured. The mistake was in confusing partnership in a bureaucratic process (putting the health agency and city council in the centre) with participation in a social change process (where the problem of ensuring policies for healthy housing are central). Instead of asking 'How can I involve community groups in my policy work?', the partnership question the practitioner should have been asking herself is 'What activities are best suited to the end: effecting political change in housing policy?' (Labonte, 1993).

This requires a recognition that her organizational requirements for change differ from those for community groups and, particularly, for activist leaders within those groups. Instead, health agencies needed to support the positions raised by local coalitions, helping to legitimize these issues by their support and by any new policy they might create.

5 Empowering communities to take social and political action

Whilst individuals are able to influence the direction and implementation of a programme through their inputs and active participation, this alone does not constitute community empowerment. The difference between participatory and empowerment approaches lies in the agenda and purpose of the process. Empowerment approaches have an explicit purpose to bring about social and political action and this is embodied in their sense of liberation, struggle and political action. If concerned individuals remained at the small mutual group level, the conditions leading to their poverty would not be resolved. If people only engaged in mainstream forms of lobbying through community organization and partnership development, without civil protest or other forms of political action, those with power-over economic and political decisions would have little reason to listen. Individuals progress along the continuum from a position of personal action to a point where they are collectively involved with redressing the deeper underlying causes of their concern through social and political action.

Gaining power to influence economic, political, social and ideological change will inevitably involve the community in struggle with those already holding power (a zero-sum situation, as discussed in Chapter 3). Within a programme context the role of the health promoting agency, at the request of the community, is to build capacity, provide resources and empower individuals and organizations. We, as practitioners, need to recognize that working in empowering ways is a political activity and one that may have to use confrontation techniques to force the more powerful to negotiate terms with the less, but increasingly, empowered. Even within a programme context community empowerment approaches may require periods of disruptive political activity before the conditions for negotiation are possible. The structures of power-over, of bureaucracy and authority remain dominant and part of the role of health promotion is to strive to challenge these circumstances.

An action research study of a Canadian health department elaborated four key prerequisites for an empowering health promotion practice:

1 Analytically and communicatively skilled, and critically reflective, practitioners.
2 Supportive peer relations and organizational norms.
3 Community empowerment oriented managers.
4 Enabling internal policies.

This study helps to illustrate some of the important principles of transforming professional power relations (discussed in Chapter 3) and the use of the continuum of community empowerment.

1 Analytically and communicatively skilled, and critically reflective, practitioners

The health promotion relationship is created between people and, through people, between groups, organizations and institutions. The health promoter is the fulcrum upon which these relationships balance. The skills necessary to an empowering health promotion practice are many, but consist primarily of analytical and communicative prowess. Analytical skills help to overcome a group's localism and its potential conservatism or undemocratic practices, and to motivate its members to political action. Communicative skills, those involving effective listening, group facilitation and respectful interpersonal relations, allow the health promoter to share his or her knowledge, and that of the health agency, without imposing it upon or negating the knowledge generated by the group.

Such a practice is not merely an exercise of technical skills. It requires an 'ethical stance', one in which practitioners acknowledge their own initial power-over and make these available to community groups. Professional power-over (higher incomes, status, organizational and political legitimacy and ability to influence the agendas of political authorities) becomes transformative when those who exercise them do so with the intent that others in the relationship accrue more power.

2 Supportive peer relations and organizational norms

The primary support the health promoter receives in this transformative process is from his or her own peers. This support requires organizational norms that value practice styles which are empowering. Not all health professionals can or should be expected to engage in community empowerment practices. Nor do community members always want to be empowered but may require, instead, direct services that are offered in caring and respectful ways. Failure to recognize and value different forms of practice at every point on the community empowerment continuum can lead to status rivalries over higher or lower esteemed practices. Supportive peer relations also requires a hand-offs approach to empowering work. Different practitioners encounter situations that exceed their discipline-specific skills or knowledge base. Peer support requires problem-posing approaches to staff meetings, team-building retreats focused on power relations and power-sharing, and knowledge development workshops in which the social determinants of positive health are analysed. An empowering health promotion practice requires organizational respect for practitioner autonomy, flexible working styles and hours, and a willingness to accept, rather than to avoid, public controversy.

3 Community empowerment oriented managers

Flattening organizational hierarchy is a prerequisite to an organizational culture supportive of an empowering health promotion practice, since hierarchy brings with it the greater exercise of power-over. Some degree of hierarchic structure will continue to characterize state institutions and even formalized community groups. Delegated decision-making (hierarchy) is necessary to the functioning of any complex group with large memberships and multiple issues/tasks. Managers knowledgeable of, if not also competent in, empowering health promotion practice are thus essential. Such managers are able to protect the health promoter when accountability to community groups, as well as to the state, creates controversy. In turn, health promoters need to understand the dual accountability systems faced by their managers: that of maintaining a degree of civil service autonomy while 'managing' the organization's accountability to higher level state and political authorities.

4 Enabling internal policies

Health agency policies, while potentially restrictive of practitioner autonomy, can also be enabling, protecting innovative practice while constraining past practices that have been disempowering. Such policies must include specific social analyses and models that recognize the 'parallel track' goals of community empowerment (Chapter 6). They should define health promotion as a practice that supports social actions around structural conditions of power/powerlessness, through the momentum created by its own internal policies to promote community empowerment (Labonte, 1996).

The basic logic offered by the community empowerment continuum can be seen in everyday life, for example, the localized actions of residents concerned with environmental threats or the wider actions of citizens demonstrating on the streets against undemocratic or corrupt governance in their country.

In Box 4.4 I provide an example of the local actions of residents in Werribee, Australia protesting against the siting of a toxic waste dump in their community.

Finally, it is important to recognize that empowerment takes on meaning in relation to specific issues around which the group impetus grows or fades as its membership changes. There is never absolute power or empowerment for communities. Rather, both only ever exist in relation to particular issues around which individuals form communities to create, or to resist, change.

**Box 4.4:   Community empowerment
by the residents of Werribee**

Werribee is a town of 80 000 people situated in an agricultural and market gardening area close to the city of Melbourne, Australia. In many ways Werribee is a typical country town with a sleepy feel to the central shopping area which is devoid of high-rise buildings and large superstores. Although the residents of Werribee had had previous experience of the introduction of unwelcome projects in their community, it must still have been devastating news when in 1996 the local government minister announced the siting of the toxic waste dump. Colonial Sugar Refining (CSR) were commissioned by the Government of Victoria to prepare an environmental effects statement with the intention of CSR becoming the implementing agent for the project.

The actions of the residents of Werribee follow the basic logic offered by the community empowerment continuum. The announcement of the siting of the dump was a sufficient emotional trigger for outraged residents to take personal action. Their focus was against the toxic waste dump that residents felt would be detrimental to the health and economy of the community. Individuals quickly organized themselves into a residents action group called 'WRATD' (Werribee Residents Against Toxic Dump). Certain individuals were instrumental in the development of this small mutual group and its rapid growth into a proficient organization. Within a period of 18 months the community had succeeded in establishing an effective campaign to raise public awareness and influence political decision-makers. WRATD employed local experts who gave weight to a sophisticated approach of information dissemination. Local support was used to establish a computerized operations centre and partnerships with local university campuses helped to broaden WRATD's level of expertise.

The campaign was carried out in a positive and pervasive manner, constantly working behind the scenes to bring about political and social change in favour of the Werribee residents. After an enormous show of strength by 15 000 residents who demonstrated against the siting of the dump and a petition of more than 100 000 signatures, CSR abandoned the project in November 1998. Participation, the mobilization of local resources, a pro-active strategy of awareness-raising and consistent legal action against CSR allowed WRATD to defeat one of Australia's biggest companies that had been backed by one of the most determined state governments. (Strong, 1998)

In this chapter I have shown that 'community' is a complex concept most usefully viewed as heterogeneous individuals who organize in groups around shared issues, interests, identities or concerns. I have argued that community empowerment, in turn, is a multi-level phenomena, an outcome and a process which can be seen to progress along a dynamic continuum.

In the next chapter I extend the discussion of power and community empowerment into the territory of health promotion programming and in particular to the tensions that exist between 'top-down' and 'bottom-up' approaches.

5   Addressing the Tensions in Health Promotion Programming

Health promoters may want to commit to the process of community empowerment, but they still work in organizations that are programme-driven. In this chapter I address how community empowerment can be made operational within a programme context. I return to the two approaches to health promotion programmes that were introduced in Chapter 1, 'top-down' and 'bottom-up', and show that although these two approaches are often viewed as being in competition – a top-down versus bottom-up tension – in practice there is no, or at least does not have to be, any conflict. I illustrate this argument with case study examples from both approaches.

I intentionally use the terminology 'top-down' and 'bottom-up' in this book because it clearly puts into perspective the way in which the tensions in health promotion programming have been conventionally viewed. The community has traditionally been viewed as identifying and communicating its own problems to top structures in bottom-up approaches, whereas the reverse has been seen to be the case in top-down programming.

Top-down and bottom-up approaches are ideal types of theoretical best practice which offer important differences to the health promotion practitioner. In Table 5.1 I summarize the different characteristics between top-down and bottom-up approaches.

Health promotion in a programme context

Health promotion programmes always entail some relationship between different stakeholders and usually follow a predetermined design for their implementation and evaluation. The main relationship is between the outside agent and an individual, group or community who receive the delivery of resources and services. The outside agent can exist within or outside the community, and can be an individual or organization that delivers the programme. For most health promoters, the outside agent is both themselves and their employers, for example, a health department or Trust, a local hospital, the municipal government or an NGO.

Table 5.1   The different characteristics of top-down and bottom-up health promotion approaches

Characteristic	Top-down approaches	Bottom-up approaches
Role of agents	Outside agents define the issue, develop strategies to resolve the issue, involve the community to assist with solving the issue.	Outside agents act to support the community in the identification of issues that are important and relevant to their lives and enable them to develop strategies to resolve these issues.
Design	Defined short to medium term time frame, budget, stakeholder analysis.	Long term without defined programme time frame.
Objectives	Objectives are determined by outside agent and are usually concerned with changing specific behaviours to reduce disease and improve health.	Community identifies objectives that are negotiated with outside agent. These may be concerned with disease and behaviours, but also with community empowerment outcomes and political and social changes.
Implementation	Control over decisions essentially rests with outside agent.	Control over decisions is constantly being negotiated.
Terminology	Also known as community-based and social planning programmes.	Also known as community empowerment, community development and community capacity-building programmes.
Evaluation	Evaluation concerned with targets and outcomes often determined by the outside agents.	Evaluation concerned with process and outcomes and inclusion of the participants.

Source: Laverack and Labonte, 2000: 256.

The programme cycle is conventionally viewed as a process that has to be managed and monitored by the outside agent; as information is gathered it is fed back to modify the programme time frame, budget, stakeholders and purpose (Youker and Burnett, 1993). The programme cycle usually includes: a period of identification, design, appraisal, approval, implementation, management and evaluation. The initial ideas that emerge from the identification stage have to be developed into a coherent form that makes sense as a programme. This is the function of the design stage of the programme cycle. It involves the specification of the programme's goals, objectives, activities, the resource inputs and expected outcomes. Appraisal is the stage when the outside agency considers whether the programme is suitable for funding and support. The programme plan and design is critically re-examined to ensure it is appropriate and cost effective. Implementation follows, and evaluation normally begins at the end of a phase or, more often, near the end of the programme.

The way in which the health issue is defined in a programme context is one of the most important issues in an empowering health promotion practice. In Chapter 1 I identified and briefly discussed two main forms of health promotion programming: top-down and bottom-up. Top-down described programmes where problem identification comes from the top structures in the system down to the community, while bottom-up is the reverse, where the community identifies its own problems and communicates these to the top structures. Few health agencies use a bottom-up approach to health promotion, mostly adopting a top-down perspective. Community development projects, even when undertaken by NGOs – supposedly more bottom-up than top down – have often been externally imposed and paternalistic rather than attempting to share power with others (Petersen, 1994).

Top-down health promotion programmes

The defining characteristic of a top-down approach is that the health agency singularly identifies the problem or issue to be addressed by the programme and orchestrates its design, implementation and evaluation. The agency mobilizes individuals, groups and organizations to address specific disease or behavioural issues. Top-down programmes reinforce an inherent power relationship between the different stakeholders in the programme, the outside agents (the health promoters) and the targeted individuals or groups. This relationship is one of power-over where it is the outside agent who has control of the programme planning and funding and where the targeted individuals or groups are expected to participate, but not necessarily to be actively involved. The identification of the programme objectives is often based on measurable epidemiological data and is biased towards a narrower medical or lifestyle/behavioural approach, reducing health to the end points of disease. Programme evaluation generally uses quantitative data and focuses on outcomes which are assessed by 'experts' often appointed by the outside agents. The top-down approach is usually designed around one specific disease, such as heart disease, and one or more health behaviours associated with the disease, for example, smoking, diet and physical activity. The programme adopts strategies such as social marketing, health education and media advocacy, which are delivered through the community as a medium or venue for the intervention. The community is in turn defined by the outside agents as a target group or population that fits within the design of the programme, for example, an intervention to reduce sexually transmitted diseases may be targeted at youth groups. Top-down programmes are generally concerned with lifestyle and behavioural compliance to certain professionally predetermined norms rather than with the empowerment of the community (Boutilier, 1993).

Examples of top-down programmes are discussed below but would include almost all health education or multiple risk factor reduction interventions. A review of papers submitted at a seminar organized by the International Union for Health Promotion and Education in 1995 by representatives from Australia, the US and Canada found that almost all health promotion goals were set in terms of disease prevention and behavioural and lifestyle change (Labonte, 1998). Similarly, the Action Statement for Health Promotion in Canada (Canadian Public Health Association, 1996), which undertook discussions with over 1000 health professionals and volunteers, summarized that most policies and practices in the area of health promotion in Canada fall into a top-down approach. The Statement advocates a shift towards policies which support the more empowering socio-environmental approach.

The successes of top-down programmes

Given the popularity of top-down programmes in health promotion it is worthwhile exploring the reasons for their continued utilization. Notable examples of top-down programmes include the North Karelia Project on cardiovascular disease (Puska et al., 1995), the Multiple Risk Factors Intervention Trial (MRFIT), the Community Intervention Trials for Smoking Cessation (COMMIT) (Syme, 1997) and the Planned Action Towards Community Health (PATCH) projects (Braddy et al., 1992).

Despite their popularity these approaches have received growing criticism for their failures and for their small degree of success relative to the resources expended during the programme. There has also been growing practitioner disenchantment with top-down approaches in health promotion (Labonte, 1998). Successes in top-down programmes have been demonstrated on a small scale, primarily in North America, with positive behaviour changes such as parenting skills and school based prevention programmes. Hyndman (1998) summarizes a considerable body of health promotion research and notes that the success of these small scale top-down programmes is their ability to have closer connections with the community, which in turn generates a stronger sense of ownership over the factors affecting their health. Small scale top-down programmes began to resemble bottom-up initiatives rather than being strongly centralized and institutionalized top-down interventions. Of the large top-down programmes, the North Karelia Project has received the widest publicity and acclaim as a successful pioneer for other projects to emulate. Box 5.1 briefly examines the basis for the success of this project; I argue that, even accepting its accomplishments, health promoters may have been generalizing the wrong lessons.

Box 5.1:   The North Karelia Project: 20 years of success

The design and implementation of the North Karelia Project in Finland are claimed to be as a result of the demands from the community about heart health risk factors. However, a closer look at the history to the project reveals that the meaning of 'community' may have been misinterpreted by subsequent health promotion programmes. An earlier project in Finland designed to reduce heart disease by replacing diary fats in milk by soya bean and butter with a soft margarine had a dramatic success. This led to further research and implementation and a network of regional branches for the Finnish Heart Association. Growing support for these interventions led to the Governor of North Karelia making an invitation to the Members of Parliament of the province and representatives of governmental and NGOs to form a pressure group. This group petitioned for state aid to reduce cardiovascular disease in the province in 1971. The Governor himself headed the delegation, which took the petition to Helsinki to gain publicity and interest and convince the government for its commitment. This is the 'community' that laid out the demands for improvements in cardiovascular disease in North Karelia, not the primary stakeholders or people living in the community but Members of Parliament and organizational representatives. The project was launched in the early 1970s as a political reaction to the health issue (Puska et al., 1995). I believe that health promoters may have generalized the wrong lessons from the project. They have focused on the topic of heart health risk factors itself and the programme activities employed in North Karelia rather than considering the political, historical and cultural reasons why and how heart health quickly became a community concern.

Why top-down programmes usually fail

A few years ago, Nicholas Freudenberg (1997), a leading US health promotion researcher, reviewed 155 urban health promotion programmes in the US. Virtually all of these would fit within the definition of top-down programmes. Freudenberg found that, with few exceptions, the programmes were unsuccessful in meeting their objectives, and usually failed to reach the dis-empowered or to even involve their participation.

Part of the problem was that the programmes addressed a particular problem, such as HIV or drug abuse, but did not address the social and economic factors that were clearly influencing both the existence of the problem as well as the overall health of the community. Leonard Syme (1997), one of the leading American social epidemiologists, similarly provides an insightful analysis of the failure of two well-known top-down programmes in the US, the Multiple Risk Factors Intervention Trial (MRFIT) and the Community Intervention Trials for Smoking Cessation (COMMIT).

The MRFIT was a 10-year programme designed to reduce mortality from heart disease in the top 10 per cent male risk group. The trial undertook a massive survey of 400 000 men in 22 cities and randomly selected 6000 for the intervention and 6000 for the control group. The trial was the most ambitious, expensive and intensive anywhere tried at the time in 1971. The trial failed and after six years the men in the intervention group did not achieve a lower mortality level from coronary heart disease than men in the control group. The COMMIT consisted of nationwide studies involving over 10 000 heavy smokers in 11 cities with a matched control group. At the end of this trial there was only a modest difference in the rate of people stopping smoking between the intervention and control groups. The trial, which cost millions of dollars and used a team of highly motivated and trained 'experts' to implement, similarly failed (Syme, 1997).

Syme's analysis of these programmes points the finger at the 'experts' as a major contributing factor towards failure. Motivation to change behaviour must come from within the community and cannot come from an expert. Syme himself admits that accepting the expertise of community (lay) health knowledge, and sharing professional expertise so that community members can use it to build their own empowering capacities, is alien to many health professionals. He agrees that providing health information (education and awareness activities) does play a role in health promotion, but that it must support the issues and problems that have been identified by the community as being relevant and important to themselves.

Marie Boutilier (1993), in her essay on Canadian health promotion programmes, argues that a key objective of top-down health promotion programmes such as COMMIT and MRFIT is to improve professional practice. She argues that the unstated purpose of top-down programmes is accountability to the funders, practice effectiveness and value for money. This focus on accountability and effectiveness to the funders detracts from what the community is trying to say, what their needs are and how we as health professionals should be addressing them. Leonard Syme (1997) goes further. He believes that most people do not change high risk health behaviours and those that do, do so for reasons unrelated to the activities of top-down health promotion interventions.

The strengths and weaknesses of top-down programmes

Perhaps one of the main reasons that top-down programming does remain the dominant approach in health promotion is that it allows the outside agents to maintain control. Outside agents (health promoters, health authorities, NGOs and so on) are increasingly concerned with the cost-effectiveness and accountability of programmes to funders as budgets are cut and purse strings tightened. The advantage of top-down programming is that it allows the agents to pre-define the objectives, strategic approach, means of implementation, budget and time frame. The agents are able to maintain performance levels and monitor progress during the programme cycle by using quantifiable outcome indicators. Outside agents often employ a project manager to oversee the implementation of the programme and a team of consultants to monitor and evaluate progress. Control over decisions essentially rests with the outside agents and the community is involved primarily to assist in implementing the pre-determined programme.

Top-down programmes can be seen as a direct contradiction to the empowering principles of health promotion practice that I have already discussed in this book. Top-down programmes, by the very nature of their design and delivery, can actually be dis-empowering, especially to those who are already socially disadvantaged and who, ironically, are often the intended beneficiaries of the programme. Such programmes can reinforce people's feelings of powerlessness by ignoring their concerns, over-riding their needs and by giving out the message that their problems are not relevant to those who hold power, the outside agents and health promotion 'experts'. Top-down programmes run the real risk of coercing the community into being involved with issues which are not a priority to them but in which they are expected to participate and towards which they are expected to contribute. Labonte and Robertson (1996) further argue that communities may expend valuable resources to mobilize and organize themselves around a programme that is too narrowly focused on lifestyle and behavioural outcomes rather than on issues which concern the political and structural changes on underlying socio-environmental risk conditions.

The early trials of the Planned Action Towards Community Health (PATCH) programmes in the US by the Center for Disease Control provides an example of some of the weaknesses of top-down programming. PATCH programmes would begin by asking community leaders about the leading health issues in their neighbourhoods. These were often expressed as socio-environmental conditions such as poverty, housing, racism and unemployment. Risk factor surveys were also part of the early planning process, to complement the 'opinions' of community leaders with supposedly more 'objective' facts. These surveys showed that heart disease, cancer and specific health behaviours were the leading problems, mostly because these issues were the only ones the survey studied. Community leaders were then 'convinced' with the data that the concerns they had identified were less important than the ones revealed by the survey. The immediate programme objectives, leaders were told, should be to promote healthier lifestyles and to screen for heart disease. The more empowered leaders simply dropped out of the programme, because it was not respectful of their knowledge or concerns. Community participation in the survey-defined, expert-led programme was often low to non-existent, because the programme did not reflect their interests. Later PATCH programmes learned from this experience and no longer required the risk factor survey and introduced planning structures that built upon the issues identified by the community. Although time-consuming, the outcomes of using a planning structure such as a committee that actively involves the community can be a strength, as the example from Australia in Box 5.2 demonstrates.

Box 5.2:   The Dalby-Wambo Health 2000 Project

The Dalby-Wambo Health 2000 Project was established by the Health Department in Queensland, Australia in 1987 and applied the PATCH model. A planning committee was formed comprising representatives from the private sector, community organizations, health professionals and the community.

A combination of data collection instruments were used to develop a public health profile of the community including morbidity and mortality, injuries and the results of screening for chronic diseases. The committee subsequently identified three priorities for health interventions: ischaemic heart disease, cancer and bicycle injuries.

An evaluation showed that four key factors were seen to contribute to the success of the programme:

1 High visibility created through a logo and media coverage of the health data supporting the interventions.
2 A positive community response.
3 Continued involvement of the committee representatives.
4 Resource sharing between the different partners in the programme.

(O'Connor and Parker, 1995: 89)

Bottom-up health promotion programmes

The other main form of health promotion programming discussed earlier is the bottom-up approach. Whilst most health promotion programmes are top-down, those who actively work with a bottom-up approach remain passionate about its potential for the empowerment of individuals and communities. The term 'bottom-up' describes the role of the outside agent as one of enabling individuals and communities to identify their own problems, solutions and actions, and to be actively involved in the programme's design, implementation and evaluation. In order to achieve this the outside agent must transform his or her power-over to a power-with relationship where the community shares and increasingly takes control of the programme. At the heart of bottom-up programmes is the empowerment of individuals and communities, the very principles of ownership, community action and control espoused by the Ottawa Charter for Health Promotion, and discussed earlier in Chapters 1 and 4.

The bottom-up approach, as community development, is frequently cited as one of the central strategies of health promotion because it has to do with building community capacities/empowerment that lead to people experiencing greater control over their lives and living conditions. To achieve these ends the community must be able to mobilize itself around a particular issue. Communities are more likely to mobilize themselves around issues that are relevant and important to their lives, issues which they have themselves identified (Raeburn, 1993). Bottom-up approaches are also concerned with geographical locality, something which top-down approaches do not strongly emphasize, for example, the family, informal groups, social action groups, recreational associations and a host of other opportunities of what Fisher (1993: 165) calls 'free space', where people can meet to discuss their needs and the issues that influence their lives.

There remains considerable confusion amongst health agencies and health promoters about what bottom-up actually means and how it can be effectively implemented. The bottom-up approach is also criticized for the absence of case study evidence which rigorously analyses its theory and provides actual examples of its successes and failures. John Raeburn (1993), an early writer on community development approaches to health promotion, recognized that some of the strongest evidence for success comes from projects in the developing world. These case studies reveal common characteristics: a small scale, usually implemented through NGOs rather than state bureaucracies, using an flexible and participatory approach. These characteristics are often alien to large bureaucratic agencies such as government departments, whose concern is increasingly with pre-defined goals and outcomes, accountability and cost-effectiveness to funders. Government bodies often employ 'economies of scale' at the regional or national level with little accommodation for feedback and re-design during the development of the programme. Here I am simply implying that bureaucratic norms are often more constraining on health promoters working in government and become more rigid the higher one goes (from local, to provincial, to national government departments).

The experience of developing countries may not be directly applicable to industrialized countries; however, the successes of these experiences have acted as a catalyst for projects in industrialized countries, such as the communal kitchens project organized by poor urban women in Peru (Barrig, 1990) and replicated in poor communities across Canada (Labonte, 1998). In Box 5.3 I provide an example of a bottom-up approach to community action in a Guatemalan village.

> ## Box 5.3: Organizational structures in a Guatemalan village
>
> Marilyn Tonon (1980) describes the community action in a Guatemalan village in order to bring about improvements in sanitation. The village was patriarchal and controlled by men, especially in regard to activities outside the home. The agents were sensitive to the cultural context of participation in the programme and did not try to involve women in male meetings. Leadership was reputational from informal male opinion leaders in the village and these people were invited to take part in discussions in regard to the project. This relatively small group of people held several meetings before itself establishing the Community Betterment Committee, consisting of 25 male community members, a community-based (bottom-up) organization.
>
> Through the Betterment Committee the outside agent had the support of the community and was able to collaborate without seeking to control or limit its activities. The establishment of the Betterment Committee followed existing community procedures, but as Tonon (1980) points out it did not become cohesive and fully functional until its members '... began to know one another, discover commonalties and assume the role of committee member or elected officer'. This process took many months of socializing and meeting as a committee, but was a crucial part of establishing a functional organizational structure within the community.

Do bottom-up programmes work?

Bottom-up programmes can and do lead to empowerment. Two exemplars of success using this approach are worthy of discussion because they help to illustrate many of the points raised above: the Alcohol Substance Abuse Prevention Programme (Wallerstein and Bernstein, 1988) and the Tenderloin Seniors Organizing Project (Minkler, 1997).

The Alcohol Substance Abuse Prevention Programme

Nina Wallerstein and Ed Bernstein (1988) analysed the Alcohol and Substance Abuse Prevention (ASAP) Programme that operated through the University of New Mexico in 1982. The Programme adapted Brazilian 'popular educator', Paulo Freire's principles and techniques of engendering a 'critical consciousness' amongst people. This involves a methodology of listening, dialogue and action by groups. Achieving critical consciousness is a slow process that may need to be facilitated to enable community members to analyse their problems and reflect upon possible new actions. This leads the community into a cycle of action/reflection/action and eventually to collective social and political activity (Freire, 1973).

The ASAP Programme sought to empower youth from high-risk populations to make healthier choices in their own lives and to play active political and social roles in society. The Programme approach brought small groups of high-school students together in the settings of a hospital emergency centre and a county detention centre to interact with patients and detainees who had drug-related problems. Youths were able to share experiences directly with the inmates and learn through asking questions and exploring problems at different levels.

The Programme was facilitated as a joint effort between the outside agents (the University) and the students who formed a Students Against Drunk Driving (SADD) chapter. The formation of the chapter was triggered when one of the students was killed in a drink-related driving accident. Gradually after more than two years the students began to take a leadership role and organized meetings and events to raise the issues of drug abuse and drink-driving in village meetings. The Programme evaluation showed that the students had a statistically significant increase in self-reported perception of the risks involving drinking and drug abuse as compared to the control group, which showed a significant drop in perception. Wallerstein and Bernstein (1988) concluded that the success of the Programme could be attributed to a number of factors including the following:

• The Programme was committed to the empowerment of individuals and communities; that was its defining ethic.
• The focus was participant-centred with the youth taking responsibility and sharing ideas, thoughts and experiences to develop strategies around their concerns.
• The programme was a joint effort between the outside agents and the participants, where the outside agents brought resources (knowledge, money, opportunities) that they made available to participants for their own use.
• It was small scale and capable of being managed by the students.
• It promoted connectedness, social support, leadership and organizational structures.

The Tenderloin Seniors Organizing Project

Meredith Minkler (1997), another key US health and community development theorist, provides a case study account of the Tenderloin Seniors Organizing Project (TSOP) in San Francisco's Tenderloin district. The Project used a bottom-up approach to health promotion in a poor neighbourhood amongst low income elders. This group of almost homeless and destitute people living in single occupancy hotels had previously been labelled 'unorganizable' by the local authorities. The group was set up by health educators and students to demonstrate that community organization can be used as a vehicle to community empowerment. The Project's objectives were to build the competencies and leadership skills of the residents to reduce their feelings of social isolation and enhance social networks within the Tenderloin district. The Project used three theoretical areas to guide its implementation: social support, Paulo Freire's principles of critical consciousness, and an approach of community organization in accordance with Saul Alinsky's theory that people come together around a shared interest or concern to take action (Alinsky, 1969; 1972).

The Project was initiated by outside organizers (outside agents) starting in one hotel to organize a core group of elderly people who met regularly to discuss their problems of loneliness, crime and rent increases. Freire's techniques were used to pose questions and identify solutions, and Alinsky's approach was used to promote social interaction opportunities to begin to address people's needs. Several other groups were established; over time, as trust and relationships developed, these groups recognized the value of linking with one another and to working on shared problems.

Minkler (1997) saw the establishment and active continuation of the support groups and tenants' associations as TSOP's greatest achievement. She cites a number of 'tangible victories' by these groups, such as organizing a protest against rent increases, lobbying landlords for changes in eviction policy, improvements in the design of bathrooms to accommodate disabled people and establishing security of tenure. Qualitative data provided anecdotal evidence of an improvement in health and wellbeing, including improved feelings of support, and reported decreases in alcohol consumption and smoking. Quantitative data was collected on 24-hour diet, recalls and the results showed a higher consumption of fruit and vegetables. Other indicators of an improved quality of life were a decline in the crime rate and accounts of personal empowerment.

The TSOP experience demonstrates the importance of basing the programme design on the needs of the community. The community and outside agents were able to negotiate and collaborate in regard to the implementation of the programme aiming to build competencies and capacities such as social support and local leadership.

Minkler (1997) admits that the TSOP success was dwarfed by the magnitude of socio-economic problems faced by the tenants. The small scale of bottom-up programmes can be a weakness unless the broader inequalities in society are also addressed. Moreover, as TSOP became more successful, it began to rely on external grants and hired its own staff. With hired staff doing more of the work, active community participation declined. When, after several years and shifts in funders' priorities, the grants were not renewed, TSOP closed its doors. This could be viewed as a defeat for community empowerment. However, it is simply a part of the longer lifecycle of communities as they organize, formalize, mobilize resources and deliver programmes on their own terms. The new organization eventually becomes its own NGO (with its own potential to begin to operate in a 'top-down' fashion), or it fades away. The important lesson for health promoters is to be aware of when it is important to help (dis-)organized and marginalized groups to create a new organization.

In summary, bottom-up approaches focus on the processes by which participants acquire new skills and a greater feeling of ownership because of their active involvement. Bottom-up programmes are mostly small in scale and implemented over a long or even undefined time frame with a flexible approach. In bottom-up programming the outside agent must be prepared to surrender at least some of the control over the design of the programme, its implementation and evaluation. This is balanced by the potential advantages of greater participation, community ownership and sustainability.

Addressing top-down and bottom-up tensions in health promotion

As I stated at the beginning of this chapter, health promotion approaches do not have to be viewed as a top-down versus bottom-up tension. Practice often moves between the two. The health promotion challenge is to work in both directions: from top-down to bottom-up, and from bottom-up to top-down approaches.

Moving from top-down programming to a bottom-up process is particularly important for practitioners such as community health nurses and health visitors who wish to move beyond 'education and awareness' programmes into more empowering forms of community practice. The logical place for this to occur is with groups they are already working with, many of which are likely to be brought together around some packaged top-down education programme. Moving beyond the time frames, content outlines and programme objectives of such programmes may be one of the more critical community empowerment moments for such community health workers. These programmes are often safe starting points for organizing to the extent that they are located in community places, and not in health agency meeting rooms which may be seen as unfriendly environments or reinforce the health promoter's power-over by being his or her working environment. Participants can even be encouraged to branch out beyond the content focus of the programmes through activities that they feel empower them and which can lead to broader issues, as illustrated in the case study in Box 5.4.

Box 5.4:   Empowering women living in low-income housing

In a low-income housing project, a public health nurse finished her six-session parenting programme. The women did not want the group to end. The nurse facilitated a discussion of other concerns that these women would like to continue meeting around: assertiveness, self-esteem, talking with their kids about sex, racism, lack of on-site fitness programmes. The nurse suggested that the fitness issue, which generated a lot of discussion, might be a good theme. It involved action, not just discussion. She also knew that the women in this group had body-image concerns. Despite all the welcoming leaflets the local recreation centre had distributed, the women would not go there. Most of the others using the recreation centre were middle-class, had expensive gym outfits and generally leaner, trimmer bodies. Because the nurse was a trained TRYFIT instructor (a programme specifically tailored to the fitness concerns of lower-income women), she offered the programme herself, in these women's homes. More women were recruited to the programme by word of mouth about where it was offered and who it was offered by; and by the childcare, transportation and promise of games and prizes provided by a local social service agency. Fitness is not the end of this programme. In the nurse's words, 'It's really only a means to an end. The end is to organize these women to improve their self-esteem and their collective control over material conditions in their lives. You start around a simple concern and it grows from there. We'll work next on racism, and on developing their own leadership skills. And we'll probably continue to work-out a few times every week, because the women find it fun and feel good (empowered) doing it.' (Labonte, 1998)

Moving from top-down to bottom-up presents an important practice problematic: the need for the professional, who often provides initial leadership in the group, to move to a position of 'equal'. Angela Kilian, a British community organizer, studied the ability of a number of community health workers to reach this status in top-down health education groups. There was some resistance on the part of many of the participating women to 'taking control'. This reflected the women's view of the groups and the health worker as still belonging to the National Health Service. One could interpret their resistance to take control as a paradoxical exercise of control against an institution they may largely distrust. As this dynamic was slowly worked through, most groups managed some degree of shift in control over the activities, but one did not. This group was the only one led by a health professional, who could not transcend the conditioned need to direct, judge and think always of group members as 'clients' (Kilian 1988). One key to unlocking power's transformative use is the preparedness of health workers and authorities to identify, and work on, those issues close to the heart of communities.

Parallel examples also exist at the level of policy work. Some years ago a Canadian city initiated an internal workplace smoking ban as a test run for a proposed bylaw. Negotiations took place between management, unions and the health department. Unsurprisingly, each 'stakeholder' had made a different claim to the issue. Management wanted to keep costs low and maintain labour peace, though they also had a concern for workers' wellbeing. Unions did not want worker solidarity split by pitting smokers against non-smokers, had a more general concern with overall indoor air quality and figured costs were a management concern. The health department simply wanted to eliminate all exposure to environmental tobacco smoke. After several months of negotiating to find the 'common ground', the issue was re-framed as one of 'no exposure to a known carcinogen', one which all three groups could support. Rather than opt for expensive, separately vented smoking areas, all three agreed to divert the funds to an overhaul of air ventilation systems and testing of other airborne toxins.

Bottom-up approaches can therefore become incorporated within top-down programmes. An example of this is given by a group of women in a poor housing project. Their concerns first came to the attention of health department staff because studies showed that welfare benefits were too low for people to meet both housing costs and nutritional requirements. In response, public health nutritionists and nurses developed packaged top-down courses on 'how to cook nutritiously on a shoe-string budget' but were disappointed to find that the women weren't interested. The women were tired of being told their nutrition problems were simply about their lack of knowledge. Instead, the women wanted, and with support from health promoters eventually created, a community garden, community dinners and some advocacy with the government to change some of the welfare policies influencing benefits. A few years later, these same women went back to the nutritionists and nurses and asked them for help in preparing and running the more packaged top-down courses on 'how to cook nutritiously on a shoe-string budget'. The important difference this time was that the request came from the women themselves who, with their increased confidence and power, were naming the issue and framing the request in their own time and on their own terms. The top-down programme had been re-orientated by the participants into a bottom-up programme (Labonte, 1998).

In the next chapter I take the discussion in Chapter 5 further by presenting a framework for the systematic accommodation of top-down and bottom-up approaches into the same programme. All health promotion work involves programmes, but not all ways of planning, implementing and evaluating programmes are empowering. Chapter 6 will identify the key differences.

6 'Parallel-tracking' Community Empowerment into Health Promotion Programming

I have so far argued that health promotion programming predominantly utilizes 'top-down' and to a much lesser extent 'bottom-up' approaches and that they have different and distinct characteristics. I have also argued that health promotion conventionally views community empowerment as a part of bottom-up approaches; but that top-down and bottom-up are not and do not have to be seen as being mutually exclusive. In this chapter I introduce a new and simple planning framework that can assist programme planners better to accommodate the two approaches within the same programme.

Top-down and bottom-up approaches are not wholly separate practices

While it is important that health promoters understand the differences between these two approaches, the dichotomy between top-down disease prevention and lifestyle change and bottom-up community empowerment approaches is not as fixed as it is sometimes portrayed. Feather and Labonte (1995) show how many health promoters, in their community work, shift between the options of marketing and managing lifestyle programmes, and efforts to organize and support community actions to change more systemic health risks in their physical and social environments. Health authorities may still keep control and may not act upon all the issues raised by the community, but the priorities are no longer the same as would be if the programme used a strictly top-down approach.

Ronald Labonte and Ann Robertson (1996), two Canadian theorists on health promotion practice, provide an example of a combination of both top-down and bottom-up approaches in a heart health project in a poor neighbourhood in Canada. Activities were initially organized as one-day community events such as picnics, fun runs and dinner parties rather than around the broader contextual issues of poverty and unemployment. Residents in this poor neighbourhood were not keen to begin on such complex problems, but enjoyed the shorter-term, one-off and enjoyable activities suggested by the heart health team. They also gained a stronger sense of their power-from-within by assisting in the successful organization of these events. Issues of poverty, unemployment and other underlying health determinants nonetheless arose in planning meetings for future activities. Even though these issues were not part of the heart health mandate, and were viewed by some as 'competing problems', the outside agents (the heart health coalition members) began to explore how they could support community members in acting on these more difficult health determinants. Although part of the heart health coalition's goal was targeting behaviour change in 'at risk' groups, they were also willing to engage in a bottom-up approach. This means that some of the concerns or issues around which mobilization and organization was to occur would be defined by the community rather than being imposed by the outside agent.

Top-down health promotion programming, as an 'ideal type' and often in practice, is a manifestation of power-over, in which the outside agent exercises control of financial and other material resources over the primary stakeholders (the beneficiaries of the programme and usually community members). It is a form of dominance and authority in which control is exerted through the design, implementation and evaluation of the programme. One assumption of top-down approaches is that empowerment can be given to the community simply through education, resources or 'expert' assistance from outside. While these may be important elements in an empowering health promotion practice, they can also create a dependency on the outside agent. Without attention to the processes involved in building empowerment, the programme often has little chance of sustainability.

An empowering (power-with) role of the outside agent, by contrast, is to make his or her forms of power-over more available so that the primary stakeholders can themselves use it. Health promoters generally do have more power or a stronger power base than the community members with whom they work, especially if committed to the ethic of improving the health of more marginalized groups. The first step towards the transformation of their power-over others is to be able to recognize the elements of their own power and to understand how this can be used to enable others to take control of their lives. Examples of these forms of professional power include health promoters' education and training, higher incomes, professional and social status. These give health promoters a position of authority. Health promoters also often have access to information and resources, can influence decision-makers, are familiar with systems of bureaucracy and may have control over budget allocations. This forms the basis of professional practice, and health promoters must understand how they can use their power to enable others to increase their own power-from-within.

Health promoters' empowering role, however, should increasingly diminish to the point when the primary stakeholders have sufficient power-from-within to become their own advocates and act on their own behalf. The outside agents may still provide specific technical assistance such as resources or skills training, but this should be at the request of the primary stakeholders rather than directed as a top-down intervention.

'Parallel-tracking' community empowerment into top-down health promotion programmes

Many experienced health promoters are already adept at merging the boundaries between top-down and bottom-up approaches. However, they also experience frustration with the bureaucratic 'power-over' tendencies of their employers, and there is little formalization of a community empowerment (bottom-up) approach in health promotion programming.

In Figure 6.1 I present a new planning framework that uses a multi-stage approach to view the tensions in health promotion programming in a uniquely different way. This framework helps to move our thinking on from a simple bottom-up/top-down dichotomy, and helps to formalize bottom-up community empowerment objectives and processes within more conventional top-down health promotion programmes. Within the context of top-down programmes the process of community empowerment can be more appropriately viewed as a 'parallel track' running along side the main 'programme track'. The tensions between the two, rather than being conventionally viewed as a top-down versus bottom-up situation, occur at each stage of the programme cycle, making their resolution much easier.

The framework is intended to be used by all programme stakeholders, but would normally be initiated by health promoters who are genuinely concerned with community empowerment and with programme sustainability. The incentive to utilize community empowerment approaches is to build capacities that can lead both to the continued management of programmes by its primary stakeholders and to increase community abilities to 'take greater control over' the important health determinants in their lives, even if these are not initially part of the programme objectives.

The issue at stake is how the programme and the empowerment tracks become linked during the progressive stages of the programme cycle.

The framework poses questions at each stage of the programme cycle to assist health promoters to identify the tensions that can exist between the two tracks when accommodating community empowerment into top-down programmes. What follows is an explanation of the main issues that occur at each stage of the programme cycle:

1   Overall programme design.
2   Objective setting.
3   Strategy selection.
4   Strategy implementation and management.
5   Programme evaluation.

Figure 6.1 A planning framework for the accommodation of community empowerment into top-down health promotion programmes

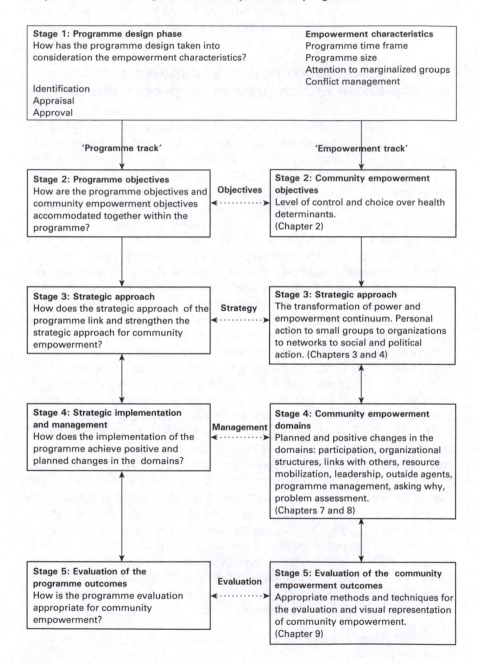

Stage 1: Programme design phase
How has the programme design taken into consideration the empowerment characteristics?

Identification
Appraisal
Approval

Empowerment characteristics
Programme time frame
Programme size
Attention to marginalized groups
Conflict management

'Programme track'

'Empowerment track'

Stage 2: Programme objectives
How are the programme objectives and community empowerment objectives accommodated together within the programme?

Objectives

Stage 2: Community empowerment objectives
Level of control and choice over health determinants.
(Chapter 2)

Stage 3: Strategic approach
How does the strategic approach of the programme link and strengthen the strategic approach for community empowerment?

Strategy

Stage 3: Strategic approach
The transformation of power and empowerment continuum. Personal action to small groups to organizations to networks to social and political action. (Chapters 3 and 4)

Stage 4: Strategic implementation and management
How does the implementation of the programme achieve positive and planned changes in the domains?

Management

Stage 4: Community empowerment domains
Planned and positive changes in the domains: participation, organizational structures, links with others, resource mobilization, leadership, outside agents, programme management, asking why, problem assessment.
(Chapters 7 and 8)

Stage 5: Evaluation of the programme outcomes
How is the programme evaluation appropriate for community empowerment?

Evaluation

Stage 5: Evaluation of the community empowerment outcomes
Appropriate methods and techniques for the evaluation and visual representation of community empowerment.
(Chapter 9)

Source: Laverack and Labonte, 2000: 257.

Stage 1: Overall programme design

The first opportunity where the top-down and bottom-up tensions can begin to resolve is in the design characteristics of the programme itself. Specifically, programme design, regardless of its content, can be made more empowering by using strategic and participatory planning approaches. Such approaches allow the involvement of the participants and help to resolve conflicts which may arise later during implementation and evaluation. In this empowering context, the concept of the programme itself changes. Rather than being a time-limited or 'one-off' educational or marketing activity, the programme becomes essentially a vehicle through which longer-term relationships between the health authority or NGO and community members are built, via the health promoter. Through this relationship, various financial, material, human and knowledge resources become available to community members. These help to enhance their capacity to act on the specific issues of shorter-term educational or marketing activities, or to organize to change specific public policies that determine deeper underlying health determinants such as housing or poverty.

Health promoters should consider particularly how the overall programme takes into consideration the following characteristics: time frame, size, attention given to marginalized groups and conflict management.

Programme time frame

It is important that health promoters appreciate the gradual developmental process of both personal and community empowerment. Several authors emphasize the benefits of having longer time frames in the design of programmes that use empowerment approaches (Tonon, 1980; Bakhteari, 1988; Rody, 1988; Eisen, 1994; Kelly and Van Vlaenderen, 1996). Other authors highlight the failure of empowerment approaches because the time frame for the programme was insufficient to achieve the long term processes of capacity building and skills development (Serrano-Garcia, 1984; Plough and Olafson, 1994; Strawn, 1994; Korsching and Borich, 1997).

Different experiences are provided in the literature for the time necessary to move from a relatively powerless to a more empowered position. Community psychologists argue that empowerment involves building competencies and can typically take five years at the individual level and, for a community, up to seven years or longer (Raeburn, 1993). Authors who take a socio-political and structural perspective on empowerment argue that relatively powerless individuals in well established communities often require only 6 to 12 months before becoming comfortable in group situations. Such groups, in turn, often require another 6 to 12 months before they are able to self-manage their internal interpersonal relations and external actions extending beyond the group.

Whatever the exact time requirement, the evaluation literature is emphatic that a long time frame is necessary in programmes using empowerment approaches. Too short a programme time frame runs the real risk of initiating healthy community-level changes that only to end before such changes have reached some degree of sustainability within the community. The result can be an increase in community members' perceived powerlessness and cynicism in the prospect of social change, rather than the opposite.

At an individual and community level, empowerment is concerned with a process of transformation through which people learn to overcome internal feelings of powerlessness and conflict and to address the inequalities that influence their lives and health. The capacities, skills and knowledge evolve through practice and personal reflection on people's own experiences. At a macro level community empowerment is ultimately concerned with effecting social, economic and political changes that improve the quality of life. Achieving policy changes governing these particular issues often takes considerable time. Moreover, community empowerment is a continuous process; it doesn't simply end one day. Not only are community relations constantly changing; as one particular policy change may be achieved, other needed policy changes will arise requiring new mobilization and action.

Longevity needs to be built into the design of health promotion programmes that wish to achieve community empowerment goals. John Raeburn (1993) interestingly argues that projects that go beyond their predetermined time frame should not be viewed negatively. Rather, this should be seen as an indicator of success because the interest of the community for the programme continues and is manifest through the ongoing involvement and participation of its members.

Programme size

Programme experience suggests that any community empowerment process should start with realistic community issues that are achievable and which can produce small visible successes in the short term to sustain interest and promote the progression onto more complex initiatives (Eisen, 1994; Shrimpton, 1995; Korsching and Borich, 1997). The programme should be designed to initially look inwards critically at interpersonal power relations and dynamics, and this can be best achieved through small groups. Later these groups will need to develop and grow into partnerships and networks if they are to effect change in their external environments. The size of a programme should allow it to be managed and controlled by the community, many of whom may have little experience and initially few skills. This can be better achieved by focusing initially on relatively small numbers of people in small programmes, thus avoiding some of the problems associated with large impersonal organizations and institutions (Gruber and Trickett, 1987; Barr, 1995).

The attention given to marginalized populations

It is important that health promoters sensitively take account of the dynamics that can affect the participation of marginalized populations in programme activities. Marginalization is a complex socio-historical process. In practical terms, marginalized groups are those who are most in need, not already able to meet their own needs, with limited access to resources or existing largely outside important social power structures. Such people are less likely to participate in programmes unless they are actively involved in the programme. This poses the question of how to involve such people in programme design and implementation. Experience in many programmes suggests that building trust with health professionals provides an important means of engaging members of marginalized groups in more empowering activities, for example, through a one-to-one counselling relationship or through empathic primary health care services.

The special importance of including women as a marginalized group has been identified in many programmes, particularly in developing countries (Minkler and Cox, 1980; Barrig, 1990; McFarlane and Fehir, 1994; Constantino-David, 1995). This is because women are viewed as being more likely to tend to the welfare, health and wellbeing of their family and, in poorer countries in particular, the education of women is seen to lead to the education of the whole family (Vindhya and Kalpana, 1988). However, the inclusion of other marginalized groups important to the empowerment of a community have been identified on the basis of age (Bakhteari, 1988), geographical location (Serrano-Garcia, 1984), caste or land holding (Ahuja, 1994) and the rural poor (Hildebrandt, 1996). The key to working with members of marginalized groups is a clear understanding of what marginalization is, and how objective material powerlessness often leads to internalized psychological powerlessness (discussed in Chapter 3).

Conflict management

Community empowerment approaches can be slow and difficult and may inevitably lead to external resistance between the powerless and those in authority and to internal conflict between different members of the group. Although conflict can be a negative ingredient of a community empowerment process (Vindhya and Kalpana, 1988; Barr, 1995; Kroeker, 1995), if managed correctly it can also be a positive ingredient (Flick et al., 1994; Flynn et al., 1994). The design of health promotion programmes should include training for the identification and analysis of potentially controversial issues and for conflict management. This can often be accomplished by activities that promote personal and group reflection among diverse members and that assist value differences to be articulated and discussed.

Stage 2: Objective setting

In conventional health promotion programming, objectives are developed during the design phase and are usually centred around disease prevention, a reduction in morbidity and mortality and lifestyle management such as a change in specific health related behaviours. The issue is how to give empowerment objectives equal priority with disease prevention objectives. Empowerment objectives are usually centred around a gain in control over decisions influencing choices, for example, over health determinants (discussed in Chapter 2) and the lives of those living in the community. The specific nature of the programme objectives will vary according to its purpose but should also be reflected in the empowerment objectives and outcomes. In Box 6.1 I use the example of smoking behaviour in newly migrated men in Canada to illustrate how the programme and community empowerment objectives can be accommodated together to be mutually beneficial.

Box 6.1: Smoking behaviour in Latin American men

During the 1980s, a large Canadian city saw an influx of immigrants and political refugees from Latin America. Often fleeing repression in their home lands, these families experienced the stresses of finding housing and work in a foreign culture, with a different language, often under the uncertainty of whether they would be able to stay permanently. They also smoked a lot, particularly the men. This caught the attention of a health department that, at the time, was flush in anti-tobacco grants money. Conventional programme objectives concerned education and awareness campaigns, designed in culturally and linguistically sensitive ways and marketed through channels, such as church and refugee assistance groups.

But community workers also knew that, until their lives and living conditions settled down, smoking would never be much of an issue for these men. Spanish-speaking health workers, still working to develop smoking awareness programmes, also asked the men about their greatest health worries. Consensus developed that it was less about them and more about their children. Their teenagers had nowhere to go once school was over and before they returned home from their sundry menial jobs. They feared that, alienated and unattended, their children would turn to the 'street life', becoming seduced by drugs and petty crime. They wanted to create a drop-in centre for Hispanic youth, with programmes that would help their kids adjust to their new world. Along with other social agencies, health workers and anti-tobacco grants money were put to work helping these men establish just such a centre.

Conventional programme objectives concerned increased awareness of tobacco-related health risks; as one example, there was no smoking during planning meetings to develop the youth centre. They extended to efforts to prevent smoking among their children, and health-related courses became part of the structured programmes in the drop-in centre. Programme objectives also incorporated the different steps involved in planning for the drop-in centre. Empowerment objectives, in turn, concerned the quality of men's participation in the planning group, the degree of leadership that arose within the group, their ability to mobilize resources both internal and external, and the extent of decision-making authority over programme planning and implementation that the men experienced. (Labonte, 1998)

Empowerment objectives are likely to change for programme participants as their own experiences of capacity and power increase over time. This 'learning-in-action' is what typifies more 'bottom-up' or empowering approaches to health promotion. Broad health concerns that might be expressed initially by groups, for example, reducing poverty in a given local-ity, may change as the group engages in activities towards this long-term goal. Through strategies such as outreach, dialogue and problem analysis, the group may decide to narrow its focus towards more immediate and resolv-able issues, for example, improving living conditions in public housing.

Stage 3: Strategy selection

It is important that whatever strategies are used by the programme they should strengthen community empowerment. In Chapter 3 I illustrate how professional power relationships can be strengthened in health promotion practice and in Chapter 4 I illustrate how community empowerment, as a dynamic process, can be strengthened along a five-point continuum. The role of the outside agents is to contribute towards this process, partly by attend-ing to the dynamics that underpin the different points along the continuum, and partly by ensuring that the strategies they use build momentum.

However, the vast range of potential strategies encompassed by all five points of the continuum are not the responsibility of any one health pro-moter, or even of any one health authority or organization. Movement along the continuum often involves health promoters working in their own inter-agency partnerships with other community workers and orga-nizations. The responsibility of health promoters, instead, is to see that the whole process is engaged, and to find their own place in its engagement.

In regard to the example in Box 6.1, this would include ensuring that individual men were encouraged to participate in mutual support groups; that these groups employed strategies to establish and build the capacities of community organizations; and that these organizations used strategies to develop coalitions and partnerships leading towards social and political change, for example, in policy and programme resources for Latin American men.

Achieving these empowerment objectives would improve the quality of their social relations with each other (social support), their collective and individual experience of capacity (self-efficacy, self-esteem, perceived power) and their perception as an important group by other institutions and social actors (political legitimacy, social status). These are associated with greater programme sustainability.

Stage 4: Strategy implementation and management

Health promoters require both the practical methodologies and examples of 'good practice' for the assessment and strategic planning of community empowerment in a programme context. In Chapter 7 I provide an interpretation of each of nine 'operational domains'. A brief summary of each domain is provided in Table 6.1. A domain is an area of influence, in this case one that influences the process of community empowerment. Positive changes or improvements in each of the domains represent a more empowered, or capable, community, one that is better able to exercise control over the determinants of its health. In Chapter 8 I describe a methodology that is designed to allow the stakeholders of a programme to apply the 'domains' to strengthen the links between the 'programme and empowerment tracks', illustrated in Figure 6.1, during the stage of strategy implementation and management in health promotion programmes. This is particularly important in top-down programming when the community does not usually determine the purpose and approach of the programme, which is as much concerned with cost-effectiveness and accountability to the funders as it is with outcomes.

Community involvement is therefore very important to ensure that strategy implementation and management is also an empowering practice. Jan Smithies and Georgina Webster (1998: 94) provide a case study example of community involvement in the Hutson Street Health Project in Bradford, England. The project covered a deprived inner-city area and was established to work on community health through a number of interconnecting ways, such as establishing networks and group activities. An evaluation of the project found that community involvement was promoted through word-of-mouth rather than through official channels. Community confidence was built up through small group activities such as cooking and exercise classes, a credit union and a play group for children.

The project was steered by the expressed needs and involvement of the community, facilitated by the sympathetic role of the health promoter, and this allowed the community to develop its own actions and activities (the strategy). The evaluation of the project showed that it had a strong positive affect on the confidence of the community members, who also felt that this in turn had had a positive influence on their health.

A second case study by Smithies and Webster (1998: 165) in the Western Isles Health Board in Scotland summarized that the effective management of a programme needs time, commitment at an early stage and ongoing multi-agency (including the community) involvement. In particular:

Table 6.1   The operational domains

Domain	Description
Participation	Participation is basic to community empowerment. Only by participating in small groups or larger organizations can individual community members better define, analyse and act on issues of general concern to the broader community.
Leadership	Participation and leadership are closely connected. Leadership requires a strong participant base, just as participation requires the direction and structure of strong leadership. Both play an important role in the development of small groups and community organizations.
Organizational structures	Organizational structures in a community include small groups such as committees, church and youth groups. These are the organizational elements that represent the ways in which people come together in order to socialize and to address their concerns and problems. The existence of and the level at which these organizations function is crucial to community empowerment.
Problem assessment	Empowerment presumes that the identification of problems, solutions to the problems and actions to resolve the problems are carried out by the community. This process assists communities to develop a sense of self-determination and capacity.
Resource mobilization	The ability of the community to mobilize resources both from within and the ability to negotiate resources from beyond itself is an important factor in its ability to achieve successes in its efforts.
'Asking why'	The ability of the community to critically assess the social, political, economic and other causes of inequalities is a crucial stage towards developing appropriate personal and social change strategies.
Links with others	Links with people and organizations, including partnerships, coalitions and voluntary alliances between the community and others, can assist the community in addressing its issues.
Role of the outside agents	In a programme context outside agents are often an important link between communities and external resources. Their role is especially important near the beginning of a new programme, when the process of building new community momentum may be triggered and nurtured. The outside agent increasingly transforms power relationships between himself or herself, outside agencies and the community, such that the community assumes increasing programme authority.
Programme management	Programme management that empowers the community includes the control by the primary stakeholders over decisions on planning, implementation, evaluation, finances, administration, reporting and conflict resolution. The first step toward programme management by the community is to have clearly defined roles, responsibilities and line management of all the stakeholders.

Source: Laverack and Labonte, 2000: 260

- a small steering group made up of people who are prepared to put time and skills into the process at the community and strategic levels;
- regular feedback to the community;

- an opportunity to reflect and act on the lessons learnt; and
- people who are 'empowered' and prepared to follow-up on recommendations.

Stage 5: Programme evaluation

The final stage of the planning framework is the evaluation of programme and community empowerment outcomes. Community empowerment can be a long and slow process. Particular outcomes in the community empowerment process may not occur until many years after the programme time frame has been completed. Thus, evaluation of community empowerment within a programme context, which has a limited time frame, can more appropriately assess changes in the process rather than any particular outcome. In effect, the process becomes the outcome. To return to the example of smoking behaviour in Box 6.1, the empowerment outcomes for the men in the group would be determined by the men themselves. Success would be judged in terms of how these men, and their families, experienced a greater sense of control over important issues, including the men's abilities to define their own project outcomes, and to evaluate their accomplishment in terms that make sense to them.

The concept of empowerment is concerned with the experiences, opinions and knowledge of people such as the Latin American immigrants and their families in Box 6.1. It is a construction of individual and collective local beliefs and 'truths'. The selection of an appropriate evaluation methodology for the evaluation and visual representation of community empowerment should account for different subjective experiences and allow these to be accessed as a part of the assessment.

As discussed earlier in this chapter, the programme design can be made more empowering when using participatory planning and evaluation approaches that involve the community. Jan Smithies and Georgina Webster (1998) provide several case study examples of the way in which community development projects in the UK have been able to draw out lessons from evaluation, including:

- the need to consider evaluation from the outset, and include funds in the project budget for an evaluation;
- ensuring that evaluation is built into the job descriptions of project staff;
- the development of skills and expertise of the project stakeholders;
- the need for a suitable local base;
- the need for a clear line management structure within the project team;
- the need for clear responsibilities and duties and to work towards a partnership with local people; and
- the need for a long time frame to accommodate measurable changes in the project.

Smithies and Webster also draw out the methods that various projects have undertaken better to involve the community in the process of evaluation such as oral history work, photographs (photo novella is an established participatory approach based on the work of Paulo Freire, and examples of using this approach are discussed in Wang and Burris, 1994), tape recordings of conversations with the community, write-ups and events and verbal feedback.

The operational domains, discussed above in 'Strategy implementation and management', can also be used to evaluate the process of community empowerment within a programme context. Appropriate methods for the evaluation of community empowerment that involve the community and apply the operational domains are discussed in detail in Chapter 9.

In the next chapter I describe the nine operational domains of community empowerment and their implication for an empowering health promotion practice, and then in Chapter 8 I discuss their practical application by using three case study examples.

7 The Domains of Community Empowerment

This chapter provides new information that can help clarify the areas of influence on the process of community empowerment. These are called the operational or empowerment 'domains' and have already been introduced in Chapter 6 as part of a framework for accommodating community empowerment into top-down programming. Here I provide an interpretation of each 'domain' and relate this to an empowering health promotion practice.

The empowerment domains are the organizational areas of influence on the process of community empowerment. I identify and discuss nine domains: participation, leadership, organizational structures, problem assessment, resource mobilization, asking why, links with others, the role of outside agents, and programme management. These domains are based on an extensive review of the community development, community empowerment and community capacity-building literature, review by 'experts', and field tested in a number of different countries and health promotion programme settings. The domains represent those aspects of the process of community empowerment that allow individuals and groups to organize and mobilize themselves towards social and political change. The organizational aspects in themselves may act as a proxy measure for the social aspects of community empowerment, for example, the existence of functional leadership, supported by established organizational structures with the participation of its members who have demonstrated the ability to mobilize resources, would indicate a community which already has strong social support elements (Laverack, 2001).

Participation

Participation is basic to community empowerment; it describes the involvement of individual community members in small groups and in larger organizations. It is a characteristic of each step along the community empowerment continuum, discussed in Chapter 4. David Zakus and Catherine Lysack provide a comprehensive and useful definition of community participation in health programmes as:

... the process by which members of the community, either individually or collectively and with varying degrees of commitment: develop the capability to assume greater responsibility for assessing their health needs and problems; plan and then act to implement their solutions; create and maintain organizations in support of these efforts; and evaluate the effects and bring about necessary adjustments in goals and programmes on an on-going basis. (1998: 2)

This definition encompasses many of the characteristics of an empowered community, essentially allowing people to become involved in activities which influence their lives and health. Roger Shrimpton (1995), an international aid worker, distinguishes between 'social participation' gained through decision-making towards greater control over factors determining health and 'direct participation' through the mobilization of resources.

There is considerable overlap between the concepts of community participation and community empowerment and the two have been included as a part of a number of frameworks explaining grassroots participation. The most widely used is Sherry Arnstein's ladder of participation, a continuum involving: non-participation (manipulation and therapy); degrees of tokenism (informing, consultation and placation); and degrees of power (partnership, delegated power and citizen control) (Arnstein, 1969). However, whilst individuals are able to influence the direction and implementation of a programme through their participation, this alone does not constitute community empowerment. Empowerment has an explicit purpose to bring about social and political changes, usually through affecting public policies, decision-making authority and resource allocation. For participation to be empowering it must not only involve the development of skills and abilities, but also a political concern to enable people to decide and to take action.

The overlap between these two concepts therefore lies in how people participate or become empowered. Robert Goodman and his colleagues (1998) address the issue of how people participate and agree in their conclusions that it is a combination of involvement in decision-making mechanisms, accessibility to community level activities (social networks, community groups, social movements, coalitions, voluntary agencies and community development programmes), and accessibility to community skills (planning, resource mobilization, organizational skills and advocating change). Susan Rifkin (1990), a writer on participation and community development, specifically discusses how people participate within the context of health programmes. Rifkin argues that this occurs at five different levels: in the programme's benefits; in its activities; during implementation; in programme monitoring and evaluation; and in programme planning. Many of these same characteristics can be observed during the process of community empowerment in health promotion programmes. In Box 7.1 I provide the main characteristics of participation as a part of empowering programmes.

Leadership

Goodman et al. (1998) also point out that participation and leadership are closely connected. Leadership requires a strong participant base just as participation requires the direction and structure of strong leadership. Leaders play an important role in the development of small groups and community organizations.

Box 7.1:   The characteristics of participation in empowering programmes

- A strong participant base involving all stakeholders, including marginalized groups, but sensitive to the cultural and social context; for example, it may not be appropriate for women to attend meetings with men.
- Participants involved in defining needs, solutions and actions.
- Participants involved in decision-making mechanisms at planning, implementation and evaluation stages of the programme.
- Participation goes beyond the benefits and activities of the programme; for example, it extends to broader issues such as the structural causes of poverty.
- Mechanisms exist to allow free flow of information between the different stakeholders in the programme.
- Community representatives are appointed by its members and do not represent élite groups.

Participation without a formal leader who takes responsibility for getting things done, dealing with conflict and providing a direction for the group can often lead to disorganization. In a programme context leaders are often introduced as external organizers because they are seen to have the necessary management skills and expertise. However, in most communities, leaders are historically and culturally determined and programmes that ignore this have little chance of success. They must at least have the support of local leaders and must also aim to develop local leadership skills (Rifkin, 1990).

Both Rifkin (1990) and Goodman et al. (1998) caution that the structure of community leadership, which may be historically or culturally determined, can exclude marginalized groups and represent only the élite. Certain groups within a community may not support the programme's aims or may be in conflict with one another. Their inclusion can create dysfunction in the planning and implementation of the programme and make it more difficult to achieve the aims and objectives. However, to actively exclude certain groups is undemocratic and does not allow full community participation. Many programmes have used a model of promoting the vision and personal leadership of one local charismatic individual, reflecting a socio-cultural tendency to follow strong leadership.

Norman Uphoff (1990), an expert in rural development, calls this 'leaderitis' and relates his experiences in small farmer development programmes in Nepal. Individual leaders dominated because they liked the power and prestige or because they thought that no one else could lead the people. The leader may be effective, but this keeps the potential leadership small and leaves the community vulnerable. Once such charismatic leaders have gone, the vision is not shared by the community because the programme does not address their needs and consequently loses its impetus. Mechanisms must exist to ensure the continuity of policy even after charismatic leaders have left the programme. As a solution to the problem of selecting appropriate leadership, Goodman et al. (1998) argue that a mix of different types of leaders has a better chance of leading to community capacity, and likewise to community empowerment.

Karina Constantino-David (1995), an expert and writer in community development, discusses the experiences of community organizing in the Philippines and the success of utilizing local leaders or 'organic organizers'. Competent leaders were developed by NGOs amongst poor people who offered a more insightful understanding of the community problems and culture. However, it was found that a lack of skills training and previous management experience of these people created limitations in their role as leaders. Leadership style and skills can therefore influence the way in which groups and communities develop and in turn this can influence empowerment.

Programmes have the potential to develop many of the skills necessary for effective leadership. Karol Kumpfer, an American psychologist, and her colleagues (1993) found that the effective leaders had characteristics such as leadership style, decision-making style, networking and visibility and political efficacy. Other leadership skills include:

- the sharing of power and institutionalizing internal democracy within NGOs and people's movements;
- an empowerment style of leadership that encourages and supports the ideas and planning efforts of the community, using democratic decision-making processes and the sharing of information;
- the ability to boost the confidence of participants and to develop in them a belief that they can succeed;
- 'transformational leaders' who have the ability to directly influence the potency and dynamics of a group; and
- collecting and analysing data; evaluating community initiatives; facilitation; problem solving; conflict resolution; advocacy; and the ability to connect to other leaders and organizations to gain resources and establish partnerships.

A high level of skills are therefore necessary for effective leadership and outside agents can play an important role in strengthening this domain in a health promotion programme context.

Organizational structures

Organizational structures in a community include small groups such as committees, church and youth groups. These are the organizational elements that represent the ways in which people come together in order to socialize and to address their concerns. In a programme context it is also the way in which people come together to identify their problems, to find solutions to their problems and to plan for action to resolve their problems. The existence of and the level at which these organizations function is crucial to community empowerment.

A review of over 150 health projects (Rifkin, 1990) found that those which succeeded in meeting their goals did so because existing organizational structures gave all stakeholders an opportunity for collaboration and support. A similar pattern in a review of rural development projects found that the successful ones were developed through existing formal or informal organizations (Shrimpton, 1995). When existing organizational structures are not present, outside agencies have utilized organizations in other fields or have themselves established committees on the basis of strong leadership.

Organizational structures such as committees are themselves insufficient to guarantee the organization and mobilization of the community. There must also be a sense of cohesion or a sense of community amongst its members. This is characterized by a concern for community issues, a sense of connection to the people (family, friendships) and feelings of belonging manifested through customs, place, rituals and traditions. Madeleen Wegelin-Schuringa (1992), a field worker in international water and sanitation, found that community members in Pakistan, India and Cambodia who had a sense of community and who were able to inter-relate to their own situation and to that of others had a better chance of establishing organizational structures. The interpretation of organizational structures therefore has two distinct but inter-related dimensions: the organizational dimension of committees and community groups; and the social dimension of a sense of belonging, connectedness and personal relationships.

In Box 7.2 I provide an example of an organizational structure that was established in England to help reduce the rate of suicide in farming communities.

Box 7.2:   Community organization to reduce suicide in farming communities

The North Yorkshire Rural Initiative (NYRI) was established in 1994 to help reduce suicide rates in the county's farming community. Suicide causes about 1 per cent of all deaths in England, with the highest proportion of deaths in any one occupational group being farmers with an average of 48 suicides per year.

Suicide is often seen as an indicator of many underlying disorders such as stress, anxiety, mental illness and depression.

The NYRI was established as an alliance between different but mutually interested representatives from the community, public and private sectors. The purpose of the NYRI was to raise awareness of the difficulties faced by farmers and the risk factors for suicide, and to direct the farming community to the help available for coping and social support such as counselling services. The members of the NYRI had to first secure support from their employers to attend meetings every two months. At the annual meeting an action plan was developed and implemented over the next year. Activities were shared amongst the members of the organization.

The NYRI identified a number of initiatives including the development of a 'helpcard' to give information on the sources of assistance in the community. This initiative received private sector support to print the helpcard and was promoted with a full media coverage and distribution to farmers, young farmers' clubs and wives' associations. The NYRI's alliance helped it to establish links with other organizations, clubs, groups and the private sector and to get involved in community activities such as markets, local magazines, church fêtes and parish councils.

The strengths of the NYRI were the breadth of its membership and the different skills, sources of information and funding that this brought to the organization. However, this also led to differences and friction in reaching a consensus of the outcomes of the initiative as people brought their own agendas to the meetings. For example, not every member agreed on the usefulness of the helpcard. Resolving these issues was time-consuming and could have led to the organization becoming too introspective, directing attention away from the real purpose of the NYRI.

Having such a varied membership also raised difficulties with selecting leaders, teamwork, communication skills and volunteering for duties. However, the NYRI was able to explore and resolve most of these issues and an evaluation of the helpcard initiative led to it being commended in a national award scheme. (Hatfield, 1998)

Problem assessment

I purposefully use the term 'problem assessment' because it is communities who identify specific problems about which they are concerned, in contrast to outside agents who usually think only in terms of community 'needs'. Problem assessment is most empowering when the identification of problems, solutions to the problems and actions to resolve the problems are carried out by the community. In order to achieve this the community may or may not require new skills and competencies, an area that can be supported by the health promoter.

The importance of problem assessment towards community empowerment has been identified in a number of health promotion programmes (Tonon, 1980; Pelletier and Jonsson, 1994; Plough and Olafson, 1994;

Purdey et al., 1994). Whilst many programmes advocate for wider participation, community involvement is limited. These programmes lose the opportunity, either intentionally or unintentionally, to involve the community in the decision-making process of defining wider problems which concern the primary stakeholders. This continues to be a major shortcoming of many health promotion programmes. Outside agencies must accept that the success of a programme depends to a great extent on the commitment and involvement of its stakeholders and that they are more likely to be committed if they have a sense of ownership in regard to the problems and solutions being addressed.

However, outside agents do frequently have new and useful information for community members, such as access to funds or technical assistance. My point is that this information should not be imposed over the knowledge that resides amongst community members themselves. Rather, a 'facilitated dialogue' between the community and the outside agents can allow the knowledge and priorities of both to decide on an appropriate direction for the programme. Problem assessment undertaken by community members can also strengthen their role in the design of the programme. Programmes that do not address community concerns and do not involve the community in the process of problem assessment, particularly in marginalized communities, usually do not achieve their purpose. In Box 7.3 I provide an example of a project that used a particular design to address the concerns of people living in a deprived housing estate in England.

Box 7.3:   The Bournville Community Development Project

Between 1991 and 1993 a demonstration project called 'Look after your heart' was run in a deprived housing estate in Weston-super-Mare, England. The progress of the project was tracked to record specific outcomes in regard to participation, knowledge levels and access to health-promoting facilities. The evaluation identified the key elements of the success of the project:

1   The project started by responding to the issues that local people in the housing estate saw as being the most important to them.
2   The project worker had an office on the estate, was accessible to the people living there, had a small budget and a clear understanding of how statutory organizations work.
3   The project received support from other local and national organizations over a period of five years and combined with publicity this gave extra impetus to the initiative.
4   The project was able to establish a network of individuals and organizations that supported its activities.
5   A structured evaluation gave credibility and further support to the project.

The major outcomes of the project were better access to health promoting facilities such as mothers' groups, a needle exchange scheme at the estate pharmacy, a local health centre and environmental improvements such as playgrounds and a secure road crossing area. These were the issues raised by the people living on the estate, and by having a design that addressed these concerns the project led to a stronger sense of 'community' and a place where people wanted to live. (Simnett, 1995: 213–14)

Resource mobilization

The ability of the community to mobilize resources from within and to negotiate resources from beyond itself is an indication of a high degree of skill and organization. Resources may be internal or external. Internal resources are those raised by the community and include land, food, buildings, money, people, skills and local knowledge. External resources are those brought into the community by its members or by the outside agent and include money, 'technical expertise' and equipment. Goodman et al. (1998) discuss resources in terms of 'traditional capital' such as property and money and 'social capital' which includes a sense of trust, the ability to cooperate with one another and with other communities. John McKnight, an influential American community health organizer, describes these as 'community capacities' and urges community workers to begin by helping community members 'map' or identify these internal resources. This helps them build from a position of strength; it identifies some of the forms of power they already possess (Kretzmann and McKnight, 1993). That communities possess both traditional and social capital is often ignored by many outside agents who bring with them the perceived necessary resources for the programme.

A review of community development case studies (Rifkin, 1990) found that it was often necessary for the outside agents to provide assistance to mobilize resources at the beginning of a programme. However, resources and control over decisions relating to their distribution must increasingly be carried out by the community, otherwise a paternalistic relationship can occur between the primary and secondary stakeholders.

The experience of many programmes has identified the ability of the community to mobilize or gain access to resources as an important factor towards empowerment (Fawcett et al., 1995; MaCallan and Narayan, 1994; Barrig, 1990; Hildebrandt, 1996). This ability may be an indication of the level of skills and organization within the community, but there is little evidence to suggest that this alone will make the community more self-reliant or empowered.

Asking why

Another important domain for empowerment is the ability of the community to be able to critically assess the contextual causes of their dis-empowerment and to be able to develop strategies to bring about personal, social and political change based on their heightened awareness. Asking 'why' can be described as '… the ability to reflect on the assumptions underlying our and others' ideas and actions and to contemplate alternative ways of living' (Goodman et al., 1998: 272). This process of discussion, reflection and action has been termed 'critical awareness', 'critical reflection', 'critical thinking', 'dialectical thinking' and 'critical consciousness'. It is a process of emancipation through learning or education, such as 'empowerment education' developed by the educationalist Paulo Freire, who originally developed his ideas through literacy programmes in the 1950s for slum dwellers and peasants in Brazil. The roots of empowerment in liberatory pedagogy ('freedom through education') is discussed further in Carey (2000).

Nina Wallerstein and Edward Bernstein (1988), two eminent thinkers about empowerment, point out that to Freire the central premise is that education is not neutral but is influenced by the context of one's life. The purpose of education is liberation and emancipation. People become the subjects of their own learning, involving critical reflection and analysis of personal circumstances. To achieve this Freire proposed a group dialogue approach to share ideas and experiences and to promote critical thinking by posing problems to allow people to uncover the root causes of their dis-empowerment. Once more critically aware, people can plan more effective actions to change the circumstances of dis-empowerment. Box 7.4 provides an example of empowerment education in the context of a women's health programme in America. This is 'praxis', the on-going interaction between health promoters (outside agents) and community members in a cycle of action/reflection/action that eventually can lead to collective social and political activity (Freire, 1973). This approach has been successfully used in a number of health promotion programmes (Wallerstein, 1992; Wallerstein and Sanchez-Merki, 1994), which have been used as examples throughout this book.

Box 7.4　Empowerment education in a women's health programme

Nancy Rudner-Lugo (1996) provides an account of the Resource Sisters/Companeras programme that used Freire's approach to develop the skills of women from the community to facilitate peer support groups to address and critically examine the issues of its members. The programme was implemented in an inner-city area in Florida that had a predominantly

African-American population and high rates of low-birth-weight babies and infant mortality. Support groups or 'mothers' circles' were formed as a forum to listen to the concerns and themes raised by the women. Women were also encouraged to openly discuss their problems and share experiences. The facilitators set problems for the women to address in order for them to explore the root causes of their poverty and the morbidity and mortality of their children.

The groups were well attended and were felt to increase cohesion in the community in an atmosphere that encouraged active listening and peer support. The participants mostly focused on their immediate problems and struggled with understanding the broader contextual issues underlying their dis-empowerment. Critical consciousness is a slow process and requires careful and patient facilitation to guide the participants into a process of reflection and action. In this way communities learn by trial and error from their own experiences and gradually gain self-determination and empowerment.

Links with other people and organizations

Links with other people and organizations include partnerships, coalitions and health alliances (health alliances are a favourite theme in health promotion and discussed further in Jones and Sidell, 1997: 37) to address community needs. Essentially, these links, or as I refer to them in this section, 'partnerships', are the fourth step in the community empowerment continuum. Partnerships demonstrate the ability of the community to develop relationships with different groups or organizations based on recognition of overlapping or mutual interests, and interpersonal and inter-organizational respect. Partnerships also demonstrate the ability to network, collaborate, cooperate and to develop relationships that promote a heightened inter-dependency amongst its members. They may involve an exchange of services, pursuit of a joint venture based on a shared goal, or an advocacy initiative to change public or private policies. Box 7.5 provides an example of building partnerships between different stakeholders in a health alliance in England.

Goodman et al. (1998) distinguish between social and inter-organizational networks both in a community and with others outside the community. They point out that interpersonal relationships and the social networks that these develop come from within the context of organizational structures such as church groups, committees, social clubs and work settings. Social and inter-organizational networks are closely linked. As Barbara Israel and her colleagues (1994) argue, these networks can lead to empowerment through greater community information, cooperative decision-making and involvement in the planning, implementation and evaluation of programmes.

Box 7.5:   The Asian women's swimming project

The Asian Health Forum in Liverpool, England identified a large number of cases of depression and isolation amongst Asian women in the area. A development health worker with the alliance held discussions with local Asian women and decided to approach a leisure centre about the possibility of arranging swimming lessons solely for these women. This would ensure privacy; for example, windows would be blacked out and the lessons run by other women. The alliance, between the Asian women and the leisure centre, was able to organize weekly lessons and to secure funding for a female instructor.

The lessons were very popular and timings had to be reorganized to avoid conflict with other pool activities and to accommodate the young children of the Asian swimmers. The lessons continued throughout the summer with about 20 women per session. Eventually the development health worker was able to delegate some of the responsibility for the lessons to the alliance and slowly their interest moved to other sports activities. The development health worker was then able to use this time to set up other alliances with leisure centres and to increase the choices available to Asian women. (Jones and Sidell, 1997: 41)

It should be noted that the idea of a relationship between equal but different partners being mutually beneficial may not always be culturally appropriate; for example, in traditional Fijian communities I found that partnerships may be seen to be a threat to the chiefly authority in the community (Laverack, 1999). Inter-organizational networks based on vertical relationships are also less empowering than those built on horizontal relationships because of the imbalances in power. This can lead to one partner having power-over another partner, for example, through coercion or consent, as discussed in Chapter 3.

Peter Korsching and Timothy Borich (1997), two American agricultural economists, describe a new and potentially useful form of partnerships directly linked to community empowerment. Small rural towns in Iowa, US have started to empower themselves by forming 'cluster communities'. Cluster communities are '... voluntary alliances between two or more communities to address common problems, needs and interests.' These small towns were faced with the same problems: lack of resources, decline in employment, loss of population and the closing of businesses and institutions caused by sweeping social and economic changes in society. In response, many communities have adopted a strategy of creating alliances to pool resources, discuss issues and plan for action. The emergence of cluster communities follows a pattern similar to the progression mapped out in the community empowerment continuum: initiation by a concerned individual or organization, establishment of meetings with other communities, formal organization, development of further links and partnerships, and an expansion of community concerns to address broader and more underlying socio-environmental issues. The clusters remained voluntary and small scale but often became legal entities, developing links with private and public organizations such as companies and universities.

The last two domains – role of the outside agent and programme management – are specific to the development of community empowerment approaches set in a programme context. The first seven domains are generic and could be applied to any community, either as part of or independent from a programme context.

The role of outside agents

In a programme context outside agents are an important link to assist communities to mobilize and gain access to resources. This is especially important at the beginning of a programme when the process of community empowerment may be triggered and nurtured by specific services provided by an outside agent (see Box 7.6). However, programme partnerships between primary and secondary stakeholders are usually based on vertical relationships that take a 'top-down' approach to health promotion programming. The difficulties of a top-down relationship are confounded when outside agents, such as consultants or experts, are involved in cross-cultural programmes. The cross-cultural transfer of skills, knowledge and resources is not a simple process and often fails because the outside agents do not consider the resilience of cultural values, the resistance of host institutions, resentment, mistrust and jealousies amongst local stakeholders (Leach, 1994), as well as the outside agent's inability to understand the existing strengths, knowledge and capacities of local communities.

However, outside agents can and often do play an important role in facilitating change in programmes by providing infrastructural support (Constantino-David, 1995), skills development (Minkler and Cox, 1980), raising the level of critical awareness (O'Gorman, 1995), technical expertise (Hildebrandt, 1996) and the provision of finances (Wheat, 1997). The role of the outside agent is essentially one of the transformation of power-over – the control of decisions and resources – to allow others to gain more ownership and control by discovering their own power-from-within.

Box 7.6:   The role of the outside agent in a health project

The Health Authority in Oldham, England established a 'local voices' steering group with the purpose of involving local people in health activities. The group was made up of representatives from different departments, community trusts and government agencies in a poor housing area. The group decided to employ an outside agent, independent consultants, to carry out a participatory needs assessment within the community whose members were canvassed door-to-door and invited to attend meetings to express their concerns. Child care facilities and transport were arranged and meetings were held at times that would be convenient to the community. Large meetings were often followed by small group discussions to elicit further information from the community about what they felt affected their health. These initial discussions led to the development of a questionnaire that was administered on a door-to-door basis by trained interviewers. This process involved a relationship between different representatives working and living in the community to coordinate the activities of an outside agent, the consultants, to provide a specific technical input.

The important issue is that the agents were able to collect information in a way that was acceptable to all representatives and that allowed the community members to take the necessary action to effect change. In this case study the issue was to complete a needs assessment that involved all groups in the community and which could then be used as the basis to gain the support and commitment of other decision makers. (Smithies and Webster, 1998: 156–7)

The qualities of an empowering relationship in a programme context would include a non-coercive dialogue in the identification and resolution of problems, lending professional status to give credibility and the use of power-over to strengthen community and individual autonomy. In Box 7.7 I provide the main characteristics of the role of the outside agents as 'enablers'. This term is explicitly stated in the Ottawa Charter's definition of Health Promotion as 'enabling people to increase control over and to improve, their health' (World Health Organisation, 1986).

Box 7.7: Outside agents as 'enablers'

- Making the programme objectives easier to achieve.
- Promoting the programme profile to funders and the public.
- Fostering the support of community and political leaders.
- Brokering new partnerships with other organizations.
- Clearly defining and communicating his or her role to other stakeholders.
- Facilitating change through activities such as skills training and conflict management.
- Strengthening other community empowerment domains.
- Facilitating involvement of marginalized groups.

Programme management

It is an assumption of this book that health promoters are concerned with programme sustainability and that the incentive to utilize community empowerment approaches is to build capacities that lead, at least in part, to the continued management of programmes by community members. The role of the outside agent (the health promoter) and the issue of who manages the programme are closely linked, because health promoters and their employers must increasingly share their control of the programme and its resources with the community.

Programme management that empowers the community includes the control by the primary stakeholders over decisions on planning, implementation, evaluation, finances, administration, reporting and conflict resolution. The community must have a sense of ownership of the programme, which in turn must address their concerns. One of the first steps towards programme management by the community is to have clearly defined roles, responsibilities and line management of all the stakeholders. The role of the outside agent is to increasingly transform power relationships by transferring responsibility to the community over the time frame of the programme. In Box 7.8 I provide examples of the empowering characteristics of programme management.

Box 7.8: The empowering characteristics of programme management

- The programme is managed by the community with limited supervision from the outside agents.
- The programme has a conceptual framework that has been developed in collaboration with the community.
- The programme management includes community involvement in decisions on planning and policy control, implementation (including financial and administrative control) and monitoring and evaluation.
- A dialogue on customary decision-making mechanisms is in place and is acceptable to all stakeholders.
- The community has received training in skills to manage the programme.
- The roles and responsibilities of all the stakeholders are formally documented.
- The community is accountable to the other stakeholders.

This chapter highlights the need for health promoters to be aware that each of the nine domains may have a direct influence on the success and failure of programme outcomes concerned with community empowerment. The domains can serve as a means by which health promotion practice can become more empowering by presenting a straightforward way to define and measure community empowerment.

The utilization of the domains nonetheless raises several issues:

- Are some domains more important than others for empowerment? It is not certain which, if any, of the nine domains have a greater influence on the process of community empowerment. Does, for example, good leadership have more influence on the process of community empowerment than the ability of the community to raise resources or to critically assess the contextual circumstances of their dis-empowerment?

- Is it necessary for all the domains to be strengthened for the empowerment of communities to occur? It is uncertain if all nine domains must be strengthened as a part of strategies to build community empowerment. Can communities, for example, progress towards empowerment without full participation or without functional leadership?

- Can all the domains be equally supported by outside agents in a programme context? Some of the domains can be strengthened in a more straightforward way than others, for example, local leaders can receive skills training in management to help build functional organizational structures. It is more difficult to develop a sense of critical awareness amongst members of the community or to train outside agents to transform power relationships in a programme context.

- How are the domains inter-linked? It is uncertain if one or more of the domains act together to support one another and if this has a synergistic influence on the process of community empowerment. For example, does participation strengthen leadership or the organizational structures of a community, and if so, does this lead to greater community empowerment? It is also uncertain what combination of the nine domains, if any, has most influence.

The empowerment domains are not absolutes. Each domain is inter-dependent with all of the others. Each domain can individually, and inter-dependently, influence the effectiveness of health promotion programmes, and the ability of health promotion practice to be empowering. It is not clear if there is a hierarchy of importance or if a combination of the domains has more influence. These are areas for further research. Nonetheless, these domains are derived from a rich theoretical and empirical literature, have been field tested in several countries and are being used by many health promoters in a variety of contexts.

In Chapter 8 I discuss three case study examples of the next step: how do we plan health promotion programmes to enhance community empowerment by using the nine domains?

8 Building Community Empowerment Approaches in Health Promotion

The previous chapter introduced the nine domains of community empowerment. In Chapter 6 I discussed how community empowerment should be seen as a 'parallel track' to health promotion programmes, regardless of their specific content. The programme could, in more top-down fashion, concern heart health promotion or tobacco reduction. Internationally, it may be attempting to improve child health through increased immunization and breast feeding. The programme could also, in more bottom-up fashion, be addressing food security issues through the establishment of cooperatives and community gardens, or seek to improve women's economic position in households by establishing micro-credit initiatives. In both instances, the programme should strive to move people along an empowerment continuum such that changes in power relations at the personal and small group levels are formalized into new community organizations and partnerships or coalitions aimed at influencing public policies. The empowerment domains that I discuss in Chapter 7 give a slightly different and more precise way of developing targets for progression along the continuum. They describe the attributes of a more empowered or capacity-rich community. Whether a programme is top-down or bottom-up, the task for health promoters and their agencies is to integrate empowerment goals into each stage of their programme cycle, based on these domains.

The community empowerment domains have been used individually by health promoters and community development practitioners, both explicitly and implicitly, for many years. Integrating these domains into a 'parallel track', however, is much more recent. First, I offer two case study examples of how top-down programmes can incorporate each of the nine empowerment domains. One of these examples addresses heart health promotion programmes, the other concerns domestic violence and both are set in the context of a developed country. While both are hypothetical, they have been built up from many examples of empowering community programmes.

Second, I offer an actual case study example of a health promotion programme in Fiji that has developed a new methodology to build community empowerment by explicitly using the nine empowerment domains.

Case study example:
Empowering heart health

Imagine a community heart health programme, one aware of the direct effects of risk conditions (poverty, unemployment) and psychosocial risk factors (isolation, self-blame) on heart health, as well as their indirect effects on health behaviours (smoking, diet, fitness). Consider how their programme planning might take into account each of the nine community empowerment domains:

Participation: Urging people to attend classroom style education sessions is less likely to attract participation than organizing events based around community members' interests. The programme organized people around what they liked, for example, outdoor picnics and neighbourhood tours.

Leadership: Developing local leaders means working with their existing strengths and providing positive rewards for their efforts. The programme used local women volunteers with good networks, cooking, organizing and child care skills to plan the picnics and neighbourhood tours. They became new local leaders for what eventually became a broader health promotion project aimed at a variety of issues, including housing, environment and employment.

Organizational structures: The programme realized that the locality lacked strong community structures, and used heart health, the picnics, the tours and other initial activities to lay the framework for a new organization. The organization would not be restricted to a heart health mandate. It may not always be necessary to create a new organization. A sufficient number with good internal processes and ample participation might already exist in the neighbourhood. If this is the case, they should be strengthened by a heart health programme, not competed against. But if there are no organizations sufficiently representative of community members, a new one should be developed.

Problem assessment: Residents generally knew a great deal about their health, but much of it remained within the dominant boxes of the medical and behavioural approaches (diseases and lifestyles). Health promoters helped to engage community members in a broader form of problem assessment, one that incorporated both capacities and problems in their neighbourhood (What makes people in this area healthy? What makes them ill?). This information became the basis of planning new activities, both short term (to keep participation active) and long term (to work on underlying risk conditions).

Resource mobilization: The programme came with some resources. These were largely tied to conventional heart health outcomes. Health promoters attempted to co-opt what they could of their own time and funding to support the broader-based organizing they had helped initiate in the community. More importantly, they accepted the responsibility of working with the new organization to attract resources for issues that fell outside the funders' ideas of what were legitimate risk factors for cardiovascular disease.

Asking why: Most people are aware of health behaviour risks. They are also aware of the impact of their living conditions on their own health. Rather than an 'education and awareness' approach to heart health information, the programme organized different educational events. These included some information on heart health and its underlying conditions. But they primarily consisted of working with residents in small groups analysing why some people had poorer health habits and others did not, why some people had unhealthier living conditions and others did not, and what local, state and national actions (from community members, from legislators and public policy) might remedy the unhealthy circumstances.

Links to others: It is easy to link heart health programmes with one another. The programme did this, but was more interested in linking the new group to those undertaking similarly broad-based, local organizing. This included brokering ties with politicians and policy-makers (especially around health-determining risk conditions) and supporting their advocacy on these issues through training and through their own health agency and health profession statements.

Outside agents: Health promoters, the primary outside agents in this programme, maintained critical self-reflection on their own roles: Were they imposing? Facilitating? Empowering? This ongoing self-assessment was supported by their agency managers, and was evaluated periodically through key informant assessments with community members.

Programme management: Over time, and as additional resources were obtained, the new organization took on more direct control over their activities. Control here generalized to the broader range of issues and organizing efforts. The health promoters and their agency did not pull away when these issues fell outside of the conventional heart health risk factors.

Case study example: Empowering the victims of domestic violence

Domestic violence is a problem faced by families in many parts of the world. Here I use the hypothetical case of a Women's Crisis Centre in a developed country to show how people can become empowered through health promotion programmes. Imagine a newly formed Women's Crisis Centre in a deprived housing estate and consider how their programme planning might take into account each of the nine community empowerment domains:

Participation: Special efforts were made to ensure that individual victims of domestic violence participated in mutual support groups coordinated by the Women's Crisis Centre. Other activities provided by the Centre included counselling, legal advice and refuge facilities. People who became 'triggered' into taking action by the trauma of domestic violence were given the support of people with empathy gained through similar experiences, as well as professional support from the health promoter.

Leadership: The programme used local women volunteers with skills such as empathy and administration to work in the Centre. These volunteers were supported by the health promoter, and received training and instruction in peer support. Over time the volunteers assumed the role of leaders who took more control of and ran the Centre.

Organizational structures: The programme ensured that mutual support groups for the victims of domestic violence did actually exist. Moreover, it used these groups to strengthen the capacities of the Centre (enhancing an existing organization). Some of these groups developed into community-based organizations, which received ongoing support from the health promoter and the Centre.

Problem assessment: The people who attended the Centre were encouraged to identify and prioritize the immediate (short term) problems in their lives. These included abusive relationships, lack of family support, lack of money and 'nowhere to go to escape the present situation'. This became the basis for the planning of activities and for the future role of the Centre. It was also the basis for the identification of the resources necessary to support this new role.

Resource mobilization: The programme started with limited resources. The people attending the Centre started to raise additional internal resources on a small scale through personal donations, fund-raising and seeking small government funding. The health promoter attempted to help the Centre obtain external funding through the shared preparation of grant applications.

Asking why: Discussions during the problem assessment led participants to agree that women who complained of domestic abuse were often viewed unsympathetically by relatives and by society. Women were also constrained by a political system that did not always support the circumstances of abuse within a relationship. The women, now critically aware of the injustice, decided to lobby their local Member of Parliament to bring about a change in the legislation against abuse and violence within marriage.

Links to others: The Centre used strategies to develop coalitions and partnerships with other local and international organizations involved in running Women's Crisis Centres. The Centre invested in a computer and Internet link with the resources it had raised to help establish contacts with other groups. The health promoter was able to assist the Centre by providing a list of suitable contact addresses of other centres and organizations dealing with domestic violence.

Outside agents: Health promoters, the primary outside agents in this programme, played an important role in helping the Centre to raise resources, develop skills and capacities, gain access to politicians and policy-makers and to support the Centre through training courses and their own health professional status, for example, by raising the concerns of the women at local government meetings.

Programme management: The programme was gradually controlled by the women volunteers who first worked to help run the Centre. This included management, decision-making, administration, fund-raising, liaison with the health promoter, other organizations and policy makers. The role of the outside agent, the health promoter, diminished but remained important in providing assistance and resource support at the request of the Centre. This was a reverse of the organizational circumstances seen at the beginning of the programme, when it was the outside agent who made most of the decisions regarding the programme.

In the context of this example, the programme objectives might aim to inform and lobby people in positions of authority to bring about a change in legislation. The empowerment objectives of the programme would aim to give women more control over the decisions regarding their status within a relationship and strengthen their competencies to organize and mobilize themselves toward influencing political policy. Programme resources might thus be used by women to organize themselves to influence social attitudes and/or to create support groups, both for themselves and for other family members. This would be achieved during the strategic approach and implementation of programme activities (see Figure 6.1, page 76).

A new methodology for building and evaluating community empowerment

I next describe a new methodology that is being developed for building and evaluating community empowerment in a programme context and provide a case study example of the experiences of using this approach.

What is new about the methodology is that it offers a means by which to transform the information collected during the assessment of each domain into action. This is achieved through using the nine domains as a focus for strategic planning such that the programme:

- improves stakeholder participation;
- increases problem assessment capacities;
- develops local leadership;
- builds empowering organizational structures;
- improves resource mobilization;
- strengthens links to other organizations and people;
- enhances stakeholder ability to 'ask why';
- increases stakeholder control over programme management; and
- creates an equitable relationship with outside agents.

The methodology does not therefore start with a blank slate onto which participants can inscribe their own problems or needs but provides a pre-determined focus through the nine domains.

The design of the methodology is based on the understanding that:

- The methodology should be participatory and have clear roles and responsibilities for all participants. Development approaches are sometimes criticized for only using the rhetoric of participation and that this can lead to the unjust and illegitimate exercise of power (Cooke and Kothari, 2001). In practical terms, participation allows the different stakeholders of a programme to express their views, share their experiences and to challenge existing knowledge claims and paradigms. Different participants may have different opinions and the methodology allows individuals to participate in an equal relationship between all parties and facilitates the involvement of each member through their discussion and interaction with each other.
- The methodology should be an empowering experience and provide a means to translate the information gained into action through strategic planning. The process of community empowerment promotes the capacity building of heterogeneous individuals who have shared interests and concerns. It engages them in small group activities, organizational structures and links with others towards an increased awareness of the broader social and political causes of their circumstances. The methodology allows the participants to focus on the organizational aspects of this process and provides opportunities for them to strengthen the capacity of their community in each area through assessment and strategic planning (Laverack and Wallerstein, 2001).

The methodology uses a participatory approach in four phases (see Figure 8.1).

1 Preparation (including the development of a working definition for empowerment).
2 Assessment of each empowerment domain.
3 Strategic planning for each empowerment domain.
4 The follow-up (re-assessment and comparison of progress).

This series of steps is not a new element of the design and is purposefully similar to the logical process used in other approaches such as the Precede Model (Green and Kreuter, 1991). The methodology also uses a simplified version of the logical framework system of project planning to provide a 6×10 matrix as a summary of the assessment and strategic plan for the nine empowerment domains. The principles for the design of an approach to evaluate community empowerment is discussed in Chapter 9.

Figure 8.1   A new methodology for building and evaluating community empowerment

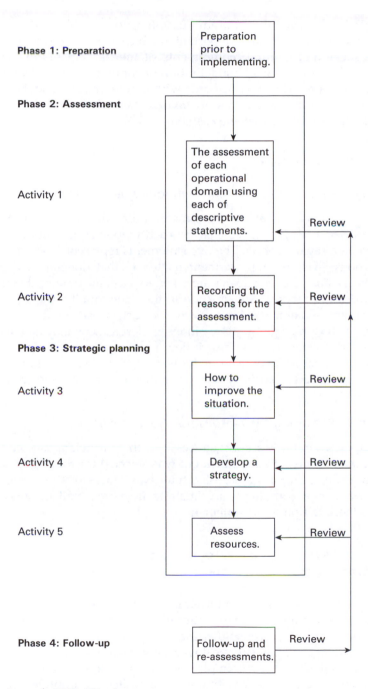

Source: Laverack, 2003: 101.

Phase 1: Preparation prior to the implementation of the methodology

A period of observation and discussion prior to the assessment of community empowerment is important in which to adapt the methodology to the social and cultural requirements of the participants in the programme. The use of a working definition of community empowerment is important to provide all participants with a more mutual understanding of the programme in which they are involved and towards which they are expected to contribute (Laverack, 1998).

Phase 2: Assessment

Activity 1: An assessment of each empowerment domain

The participants first make an assessment of each domain. To do this they are provided with five statements for each empowerment domain, each written on a separate sheet. The five statements represent a description of the various levels of empowerment related to that domain. Taking one domain at a time, the participants are asked to select the statement that most closely describes the present situation in their community. The statements are not numbered or marked in any way and each is read aloud by the participants to encourage group discussion. The descriptions may be amended by the participants or a new description may be provided to describe the situation for a particular domain. In this way the participants make their own assessment for each domain by comparing their experiences and opinions.

Activity 2: Recording the reasons for the assessment

It is important in these assessment sessions that participants discuss and record the reasons why the statement was selected for the assessment of each domain, using examples of actual experiences of the participants taken from their community to illustrate in more detail the reasoning behind the selection of the statement.

Phase 3: Developing a strategic plan for community empowerment

The assessment in Phase 2 is in itself insufficient to empower the participants, who must also have the ability to transform this information into action in regard to decisions that influence their lives. This is achieved through strategic planning for positive changes in each of the nine empowerment domains using three simple steps: a discussion on how to improve the present situation; the development of a strategy to improve upon the present situation; and the identification of any necessary resources.

*Activity 3: A discussion on how
to improve the present situation*

Following the assessment of the domain the participants will be asked to decide as a group how this situation can be improved in their community. If more than one statement has been selected, the participants should consider how to improve each situation. The purpose is to identify the broader approaches that will improve the present situation and provide a lead into a more detailed strategy. If the participants decide that the present situation does not require any improvement, no strategy will be developed for that particular domain.

*Activity 4: Developing a strategy
to improve the present situation*

The participants are next asked to consider how, in practice, the present assessment can be improved. The participants develop a more detailed strategy based on the broader approaches identified in Table 8.1, Column 4 by:

- identifying specific activities;
- sequencing activities into the correct order to make an improvement;
- setting a realistic time frame including any significant benchmarks or targets; and
- assigning responsibilities to complete each activity within the time frame.

Activity 5: Assessing resources

The participants assess the internal and external resources that are necessary and available to improve the present situation, for example, technical assistance, equipment, land, finance, training. This includes a review of locally available resources and resources provided by an outside agent.

Phase 4: Follow-up and re-assessments

It is the responsibility of the facilitator to provide a copy of the completed matrix to the other workshop participants. The matrix is the basis for further discussion, planning and action by the participants who must meet to review the assessment and strategic plan that they have developed every three to six months.

Case study example: Experiences of empowering rural Fijian communities

The next case study illustrates the experiences of a health promotion programme that has implemented this new methodology to build community empowerment in traditional rural communities in Fiji (Laverack, 2003).

Fijian villages provide a geographical boundary for the community and these are grouped into districts (*tikina*), the districts into provinces, and the provinces into administrative divisions. The *tikina* typically represents three or four communities who share the same needs and interests, a cluster concept similar to that already discussed in Chapter 7 and developed by Korsching and Borich (1997).

The methodology was implemented in two rural Fijian *tikinas*: the Tikina Health Committee (THC) of Nasikawa (involving 17 people), and Bemana (involving 14 people) on the main island of Viti Levu. Nasikawa is a two-hour drive along a dirt track from the south-west coastal town of Sigatoka, and Bemana is the neighbouring *tikina* to Nasikawa. The THC is made up of community representatives, clan chiefs and government staff from the villages that exist within the geographical boundary of the *tikina*.

The methodology was implemented with the support of the AusAID, Fiji Trilateral Health Promotion Project between July 1997 and August 1998. The methodology used a workshop approach and the assessment and strategic planning for community empowerment was completed at the community level. The following is a brief account of the experiences of the usefulness of the methodology.

The Nasikawa Tikina Health Committee: A 'kick start' response

The workshop had provided a 'kick start' for subsequent community activities; for example, the participants had developed a checklist of indicators for a safe and hygienic community based upon their discussion of the domain 'organizational structures' during the workshop. The THC members now periodically visited other communities to check for health and safety standards according to the checklist and directed remedial work to clean the environment and to repair water and sanitation facilities.

The methodology had engaged the participants in a process of logical thinking and critical self-assessment. Murray and Graham (1995) describe a similar phenomenon in Scottish communities where a participatory process was observed to facilitate changes and action after identifying the needs and resources to address concerns about local transport and the security of children's play areas. The methodology in Fiji had acted as a 'trigger' for further action involving individuals in small group meetings, establishing links between communities and raising resources to carry out the remedial work. This is a process of empowerment and capacity building along a dynamic continuum as I have discussed in Chapter 4.

Table 8.1   **Matrix configuration to improve leadership in Bemana Tikina Health Committee**

Column 1 Domain	Column 2 Assessment	Column 3 Reasons why	Column 4 How to improve	Column 5 Strategy	Column 6 Resources
Leadership Veiliutaki	Leadership lacks skills and outside support.	Have not received skills training. A lack of role identification by leaders. Inadequate support for their needs as leaders.	Skill training for leaders. Clarify role of leaders. Improve channels of communication between leaders and community. Improve networking.	Training programme for leaders. Regular meetings by *Tikina* council. Regular visits to meetings by leaders to discuss issues raised.	Training support from outside agent. Funds or transportation for leaders to reach community.

Source: Laverack, 2003: 103.

The Bemana Tikina Health Committee: Positive action

The THC was willing to openly identify that leadership was weak and that this was mainly due to poor capacity, support and communication between the leaders, the community and organizations outside the *tikina*. The participants were able to identify a number of realistic solutions to these weaknesses (see the matrix for domain 'leadership' in Table 8.1).

Following the implementation of the methodology, and at the request of the THC, a Fijian NGO had organized leadership training to address the issue of conflict resolution between clan leaders. The methodology had assisted in strengthening leadership, building links in the community, promoting participation and gaining support from an outside agency. These are examples of the domains, discussed earlier in Chapter 7, that can strengthen the process of capacity building and empowerment.

Common themes for successful implementation

The common themes for the successful implementation of the methodology were identified as: a free flow of information between participants (access to the matrix, sharing of information between the participants and with other communities and clear expectations); and the need for follow-up and support (from the facilitator and from the outside agents).

A free flow of information:
sharing ideas and visions

The need for dialogue, the free flow of information and open communication between the participants is essential for effective implementation. To avoid misunderstandings, the expectations of using the matrix must be clearly defined by the participants and a consensus reached at the time of the workshop. The expectations must be documented and a copy should be sent to the participants along with the completed matrix.

The need for the free flow of information has also been identified as an important element in the process of community empowerment in the context of development programmes by other authors. MaCallan and Narayan (1994) identify active inter-agency collaboration and effective communication as important elements. Speer and Hughey (1995) identify dialogue between the community organization and the individual as being the most important action towards community empowerment.

The sharing of information from one person to others, even when everyone had an equal sense of ownership, did present a challenge during the implementation. Traditional protocol was offered by the participants as one of the main reasons for the failure to communicate information. Traditional protocol is followed when the approval of the village chief is obtained to hold a meeting, prior to the agreement of the THC.

A chief is always accorded the outward signs of respect and thus he is seen to be the leader. Matters of tradition or culture are his concern and this would include holding meetings with the other village leaders. Even though a person may gain prominence, respect and authority within the community because of his or her personal qualities or through the acquisition of wealth, he or she would have to defer to the chief on matters of tradition and culture. Individuals may be reluctant to defer to the chief to ask for a particular favour, such as organizing a meeting, if he or she lacks respect for the chief or if he or she is not on good terms with the chief at the time. This alone may have been reason enough to dissuade the person receiving the matrix from organizing a meeting.

The need for follow-up:
fostering encouragement and support

Leonard and Leonard (1991) point out that many years of training experience in Fiji has identified the need for follow-up by someone who has an understanding of the purpose and function of the workshop. They stress that this is particularly important at the village and *tikina* levels and suggest that follow-up should take the form of regular meetings to help people to identify and solve issues which may be hindering progress.

The person(s) designated to follow-up may be an outside agent or community member/facilitator. The purpose of the follow-up meetings is to provide advice and encouragement and to resolve barriers to the successful implementation of the matrix. Framework systems have been successfully employed as a part of training in Fiji at the community level, and support to the Bemana THC by an outside agent was greatly assisted by the matrix which provided a concise summary of planned future action in the community.

The use of the methodology in this case study has demonstrated:

- that implementation was shown to differ according to the level of communication, support and follow-up between the participants;
- the ability of the participants to complete each phase as a sequence: preparation, assessment, strategic planning and follow-up. This was an indication of a high degree of logical thinking and of organizational skills of the participants;
- that the development of a strategic plan for community empowerment can be achieved in a one- or two-day participatory workshop setting; and
- that the completed matrices presented achievable, realistic and often innovative outcomes towards community empowerment.

The case study also demonstrated the need for cultural considerations to be taken into account during the implementation of the methodology; for example, the design has to be flexible enough to accommodate variable time frames, different patterns of participation, perceptions of time and specific cultural protocol.

By using approaches, as outlined in this chapter, that promote community empowerment to build capable communities as a part of health promotion programmes, we as practitioners can enable people to gain a better understanding of the problems and solutions to the problems that influence their health and lives.

In the next chapter I discuss appropriate methods for the evaluation and visual representation of community empowerment in health promotion programmes.

9 Evaluating Community Empowerment Approaches

In Chapter 8 I provided three examples of how a health promotion programme might incorporate the empowerment domains. Planning an empowerment parallel track is a two-step operation. Health promoters and their agencies need first to be conscious of, and intentional in, using their programmes to increase desired capacities in each of the nine empowerment domains. By desired capacities, I mean changes that community members think are important, and that the programme might be able to assist in developing. This requires a second step in planning, one in which community members involved in the programme in its early days participate in a process to assess what they think are their community's empowerment needs and how the programme might meet them. This planning phase is intimately connected to the evaluation of the empowerment process itself.

Before turning to some suggestions for the evaluation of community empowerment I want to briefly discuss:

- the literature on empowerment evaluation; and
- different measures of an empowering health promotion practice and some ethical and methodological points about the evaluation.

Empowerment evaluation

The main advocate for empowerment evaluation has been Professor David Fetterman, and his co-edited book defines and sets out the vision of empowerment evaluation (Fetterman et al., 1996). Fetterman et al. (1996: 4) define empowerment evaluation as the '... use of evaluation concepts, techniques, and findings to foster improvement and self-determination'. Fetterman et al. argue that although targeted at disenfranchised individuals and organizations, the approach can also be applied to communities and societies. Fetterman et al. (1996: 5) point out that the purpose of the approach is to '... help people help themselves and improve their programmes using a form of self-evaluation and reflection'. To achieve this the approach uses both qualitative and quantitative techniques in group activities as an ongoing process of internalized and institutionalized evaluation.

Fetterman et al. (1996) view empowerment as both a process and an outcome and identify indicators for the community level: evidence of pluralism; organizational structures; and accessible community resources. The emphasis of the approach is very much on self-determination targeted at the disenfranchised in a world where power cannot be given but must be gained or taken by people. Fetterman et al. also view the tension as a bottom-up versus a top-down dilemma for practitioners.

The idea of empowerment evaluation has its origins in the work of community psychology and participatory evaluation in industrialized countries, championed by such authors as Julian Rappaport, Marc Zimmerman and Barbara Israel. Fetterman et al. point out that their own work in the areas of school reform movements and people with disabilities in America have been a major influence on the idea of empowerment evaluation. This work formed the theoretical foundation for self-determination, which in turn has become the basis for the idea of empowerment evaluation.

Empowerment evaluation is used specifically in a programme context and Fetterman et al. (1996) outline the steps of empowerment evaluation:

1 Taking stock of the programme's weaknesses and strengths.
2 Establishing goals for future improvement.
3 Developing strategies to achieve the goals.
4 Determining the type of evidence required to document credible progress toward their goals.

Not all programme evaluators agree with Fetterman and his colleagues, noting that there are times of real power struggle between different stakeholders (funders, communities) that can prevent such an approach from working (Patton, 1997) and the need to ensure that such a participatory approach to evaluation does not simply provide the answers that participants want to hear (Stufflebeam, 1994).

Other authors have also suggested the use of predetermined indicators which can be utilized as a part of external assessments of a programme (Labonte, 1994; Barr, 1995; IRED, 1997). These outcome indicators cover a range of social, political and economic factors relating to the level of control, and hence power, that a community has over the influences on their lives. In a similar way, Friedmann (1992), Phillips and Verhasselt (1994) and Craig and Mayo (1995) discuss empowerment outcomes in broad contextual terms addressing the theoretical issues of power. Laverack and Wallerstein (2001) discuss the key theoretical and practical questions in regard to the measurement of community empowerment. However, none of these authors discuss the development of a practical methodology or 'tool' for the measurement of community empowerment.

Of the other levels of analysis of empowerment it has been psychological empowerment that has received the most attention in terms of developing a practical 'tool' for its measurement. Rissel et al. (1996a) and Rissel, et al. (1996b) discuss a practical methodology for the measurement of psychological empowerment, Zimmerman discusses the measurement of perceived control in relation to psychological empowerment (Zimmerman and Rappaport, 1988; Zimmerman and Zahniser, 1991) and Hayes (1994) discusses indicators of the personal empowerment of employees to determine the level of organizational empowerment.

Measures of an empowering health promotion practice

There are three differing types of indicators that are useful and may be necessary for health promotion evaluation: population health indicators, programme specific indicators, and community empowerment indicators. I describe briefly the first two of these, population health and programme specific indicators, and then go on to discuss how community empowerment indicators might be established and used for evaluation.

Population health indicators

Population health indicators are measures of important health determining characteristics in social, economic and physical environments, positive and negative health status and health behaviours. Such indicators, in effect, would be measures for the various risk conditions, psychosocial risk factors, behavioural risk factors, physiological risk factors and health outcomes defined in Figure 2.1 (see page 26). Most of the indicators of these determinants are available through statistical information routinely collected by various government departments, such as health, education and finance, or through periodic health, labour market or other surveys. These indicators are most effective for monitoring desired and undesired changes in the health of people and place. They provide a base-line from which new programme and policy development might be launched and actions initiated.

Indicators of the category 'risk conditions' also represent the development outcomes to which health promotion programmes ought to contribute. Establishing cause/effect between such outcomes and health promotion programmes is often hard to establish for several reasons:

- There are too many other potential causes in the environment besides the health promotion programme.
- Controlling for these other factors can be very difficult.
- Most programmes are too modest in their scale to expect them to have independently significant impacts on such outcomes as poverty rates or environmental pollution.
- The absence of positive change in these indicators at the aggregate (community or state-wide average) level may hide very positive

changes amongst a smaller group of people who actively participate in and benefit from the programme. (Labonte, 1998)

At the same time, it is important that health promoters develop an evidence-based argument for how or why they, and community members, think their health promotion programmes are making some positive contribution towards improvements in risk conditions. Working from the analytical framework of health determinants (Figure 2.1) makes this easier to do. So does incorporating an empowerment parallel track in their programmes (Figure 6.1, see page 76).

Programme specific indicators

Programmes require their own indicators based upon their more narrowly focused goals and objectives. These indicators are likely to reflect the behavioural risk factors in Figure 2.1, although mental health promotion programmes might well have objectives related to the category of psychosocial risk factors. More ambitious bottom-up programmes may target changes in risk conditions. What distinguishes programme specific indicators from population health indicators is that this group of measures is tied directly to what the programme intends to change. Programmes need to document the changes they bring about, especially those that are consistent with their aims (goals/objectives). To most funders, health agencies and practitioners, these changes are usually defined as 'the ends'. I suggest they now be considered means as well as ends. Community empowerment becomes an end separate to those defined for particular programmes. It exists as a parallel track to the programme itself, requiring its own conceptualization and measurement.

Evaluation that empowers

Before turning to how indicators for community empowerment domains might be established, I want to address how evaluations can be undertaken in ways consistent with empowerment goals. The four steps of empowerment evaluation discussed earlier, proposed by Fetterman et al. (1996), stand as good ideals for an approach to evaluation that, if not directly empowering, at least does not contradict the empowerment goals of a parallel track. The shortcomings of the approach (how can people be 'objective' in their self-assessments of changes brought about by their programmes?) can be overcome by 'triangulation'. Triangulation refers to use of a variety of quantitative and qualitative methods, and a number of evaluators each with differing points of view, to evaluate the same change (Scriven, 1997; Sechrest, 1997; Labonte and Robertson, 1996).

All persons involved in evaluation that at the same time empowers the participants need to share certain ethical commitments, summarized by Labonte and Robertson (1996) and Wadsworth and McGuiness (1992) as:

- Respect for all parties as equal yet possessing different values, concerns and meanings, all of which are equally important.
- A determination to seek all parties' perceptions.
- An opportunity for all to discuss and interpret the findings in order to reach a consensus on the best explanation.

Measuring community empowerment

The key points for the design of a methodology to measure community empowerment have already been discussed in this book and include the following:

- The concept of 'community' may be interpreted as heterogeneous individuals and groups who share common interests and needs and who are able to mobilize and organize themselves towards social and political change.
- Viewing community empowerment as a process along a continuum provides insight into the measurement of the competencies and capacities developed towards social and political change within the time frame of most programmes.
- The nine domains of community empowerment present a straight-forward way to define and measure this construct as a process.
- The evaluation methodology should be participatory and have clear roles and responsibilities for all stakeholders.
- The methodology should be an empowering experience and provide a means to translate the information gained into action through strategic planning.

(Laverack and Wallerstein, 2001).

These principles are sound, but what do they mean in practice? The first point I wish to make here is that there are many potential ways in which community empowerment, and changes in the nine empowerment domains, might be evaluated. The approach I describe below is only one, albeit one that has been or is being, applied in different programme contexts: Fiji (Laverack, 1999; 2003); Nepal (Gibbon, 1999); Canada (Bell-Woodard, 2002; Jeffery, 2001); New Zealand (Duignan et al., 2001); and the Kyrgyz Republic (Jones, 2002). The experiences of its practical application in Fiji has been outlined in Chapter 8.

Methods for measurement

Methods for assessing change in the empowerment domains are multiple: key informant interviews, focus groups, surveys, programme plans, other forms of documentation (practitioner logs, minutes of meetings).

Alternatively there are other opportunities to gather information such as using socio-grams (a technique to visually map or graph relationships, often used as a programme element) to measure changes in social support and networks over time. Such techniques may be part of the programme itself, as well as being sources of information for evaluating change (Have the socio-grams changed? Have the networks increased in density and resource flow?). Incorporating such techniques into programme activities fits well with the ethic of community empowerment; indeed, such techniques can help in engendering critical consciousness, pertinent to the empowerment domains of problem assessment and asking why.

Determining the rank

The three main community empowerment/capacity building models that have moved into measurement all suggest some form of ordinal ranking (Laverack, 1999; Bopp et al., 1999; Hawe et al., 2000). Michael Bopp and his colleagues (1999), working primarily with Canadian rural communities and First Nations (indigenous peoples), provide numerous prompting questions to guide assigning a summative rank for each domain. Penny Hawe and her colleagues (2000), whose work is based on Australian health authorities and community health centres, provide a number of statements that require independent ranks, though the elements of their domain and how they should be scored are still being field-tested.

I used a rating scale (called Empowerment Assessment Rating Scales) in three rural Fijian communities on the main island of Viti Levu (Laverack, 1999; 2003). The purpose was to provide a focus for the participants on each of the nine domains to identify problems and then solutions towards building community capacity. Each scale consisted of five items that ranged from the least to the most empowering situation. Each item was expressed as a short statement derived from community discussion and the literature, and a ranking was made from 1 (unacceptable) to 5 (most satisfactory). The participants were asked to discuss the five statements for each domain and to select the one that most closely described the current situation in their community. For example, for participation the ranking descriptors were:

1   Not all community members and groups are participating in community activities and meetings.
2   Community members are attending meetings but not involved in discussion and helping.
3   Community members involved in discussions but not in decisions on planning and implementation; limited to activities such as voluntary labour and financial donations.
4   Community members involved in decisions and planning and implementation; mechanisms exist to share information between members.

5   Participation in decision-making has been maintained; community members involved in activities outside the community.

This is a useful improvement over wholly subjective rankings, especially if the intent is to monitor changes in the domains over time. Otherwise, how would one interpret the assigned scores? It also has problems. During the field-testing in Fiji my pre-quantified scales were found to influence unacceptably the behaviour and actions of the participants. The use of the rating scales led to the introduction of subject bias such that they did not allow an independent assessment to be made by the participants.

The rating scales were subsequently removed and the design adapted to utilize an approach in which the participants are provided with the five statements, each written on a separate sheet of paper. In the field test each statement was written in English with a translation in Fijian. They were not numbered or marked in any way. Each statement represented an item of the range between the least to the most empowering situation, and this pattern of having five alternatives was repeated for each domain. Participants discussed each statement in turn and made a selection of the one that most closely described the current situation in their community.

They repeated this pattern for each domain, with an emphasis placed on sharing experiences and knowledge. The statements could be amended or a new statement written by the participants to describe the situation in their community. Participants could discard some of the statements and spend time discussing others before reaching a consensus about any one statement. Participants had no difficulty creating brief descriptors for each of the domains that were significant to their programme. In other cases, participants struggled initially. Participants were free to add or subtract domains that were not relevant (providing they gave a good reason for doing so), and to change both the wording and the ordering of the ranks for the domains they used.

Assigning the rank

My experiences underscore the importance of a 'facilitated dialogue' or workshop approach to assessing community capacity domains. Some evaluators who use this ranking method assign the rank on the basis of repeat interviews with community leaders/informants (Bjaras et al., 1991; Eng and Parker, 1994). Others, including myself, believe it is better and more consistent with empowerment that the health promoter and community members should assign the rank cooperatively, either as part of the workshop methodology (Laverack, 1999; Bopp et al., 1999) or, as is being used in an application of the parallel track in Canada (Labonte et al., 2002), through e-mail and the Internet. There is no simple guide for choosing which community members to invite into this early part of the empowerment process, or when to workshop the rankings. However, involving the same people in assigning ranks at different points in time is preferred if the ranks will be used to assess change over time.

Validating the rank

'Validity' in evaluation generally means that the measure (indicator) is capturing something real and unique. With reference to community empowerment, the validity of the ranking is strengthened if multiple assessors are involved (that is, the health promoter and community members), if they work towards consensus in the rank, and if they are required to offer some defense for the rank (for example, if they assign a rank of 3 for participation, they give some examples of why this is the case). The validity of the rank is also strengthened if community members who know about the programme and are familiar with community dynamics, but are not involved in the programme themselves, are also asked as 'key informants' to assess the relevance of the empowerment domains. This provides an 'outside' assessment as a check against the desire of participants to rate changes in the empowerment domains more favourably than might be the case.

The subjectivity of community empowerment, despite defining it more precisely as a function of nine empowerment domains, reflects a dilemma common to social indicators. Objective indicators, such as those for health-determining risk conditions, represent expert opinion that may not be shared by community members. Subjective indicators, or people's perceptions of such conditions and outcomes, may reflect the well-known tendency of persons living under objectively awful conditions to think that things are not that bad (Hancock et al., 1999). Including both types of indicators in an evaluation scheme allows engaged community members to question any apparent disagreement between themselves. This questioning is another example of the 'asking why' empowerment domain, the results of which provide useful evidence in programme evaluation.

It is important that the participants record the reasons justifying the assessment for each selected domain. First, it assists other people who make the re-assessment and who need to take the previous record into account. Second, it provides some defensible or empirically observable criteria for the selection. This overcomes one of the weaknesses in the use of qualitative statements or 'mini-stories', that of reliability over time or across different participants making the assessment (Uphoff, 1991). The justification needs to include verifiable examples of the actual experiences of the participants taken from their community to illustrate in more detail the reasoning behind the selection of the statement.

Work-shopping the ranking scheme

The workshop methodology recommended for evaluating empowerment domains is, essentially, a planning meeting in which health promoters and key community representatives meet to reach agreement on:

- The empowerment domains. Do they understand them? Do they capture an important quality for that community? Is the description of the domain relevant? Working in an inter-cultural context (European–Fijian), I found that considerable prior effort was needed to determine conceptual equivalencies. This does not render the empowerment domains something that changes with each group or context. The addition, deletion or amendment of a domain needs some well-defended argument.
- Order the descriptors into a ranking scheme.
- Discuss where their community ranks at that point in time, providing reasons why the rank is assigned. Differences might arise at this point, and obtaining a consensus rank may be difficult. Subtle power relations within the group can distort individuals' personal preferences to a forced agreement. These are part of any group process and can be managed with good group facilitation skills.
- Discuss where the community should be and, in broad terms, some actions that could begin to move it in the desired direction.
- Identify resources required to take actions, including the health promotion programme as a potential resource.

I used a matrix approach for mapping community empowerment and programme responses in Fiji. An example of the matrix configuration for two domains for the Naloto Tikina Health Committee is provided in Table 9.1. Marion Gibbon's (1999) work also found that the use of a matrix can facilitate the participants' understanding and discussion of the situation, the strengths, weaknesses and areas that need improvement.

The information this workshop process creates can then be used to plan the health promotion programme and poses the simple question 'How can the programme help to increase the community's desired changes in capacity in each of the empowerment domains?' The same rating workshop group and additional outside assessors can repeat the assessment from time to time over the programme life. The questions for the programme then become: 'How has the programme helped to improve capacity in a given domain (and how do we know this, what other documentation or evidence can we cite)?' and 'How can the programme improve it even further?

Using visual representations of the rank

The empowerment ranks can be used to evaluate how well the programme is contributing to desired changes in the different domains. Several authors have used visual representations to map community changes. Roughan (1986) developed a wheel configuration and used rating scales to measure three areas: personal growth, material growth and social growth for village development in the Solomon Islands. The rating

Table 9.1   Matrix configuration for the Naloto Tikina Health Committee

Domain	Assessment	Reasons why	How to improve	Strategy	Resources required
Resource mobilization *Na kena vakayagataki na i yau bula*	Community has increasingly supplied resources but no collective decision about distribution. Resources raised have had limited benefits.	People have given resources for planned activities but these were not carried out. Resources continue to be requested from the community.	Considerable resources need to be raised by the community. Community should decide on the distribution that should be carried out fairly.	A clear plan of action to include policy of accountability Regular meetings. Provide feedback from meetings to community. Leadership and management training to set a good example.	Year planner. Meeting place and small funds to hold meeting. Time frame for meetings. Skills training to leaders.
Participation *Vakaitavill Cacaka vata*	Not all community groups are participating in activities and meetings such as women, youth groups. Personal differences divide the community.	There is a lack of knowledge, skills, focus and interest in the community.	Use traditional protocol, chiefly leadership and *matagali*. Have a clear directive on the course of action.	Develop directive with time frame, activities, responsibilities in follow-up meetings.	Human resources to develop directive. Commitment to implement.

Source: Adapted from Laverack, 1999: 244–5.

Figure 9.1   The 'spider web' configuration

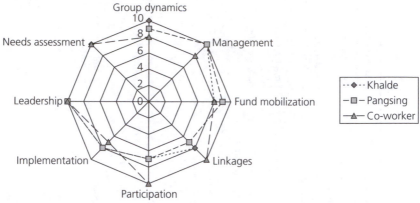

Source: Gibbon et al., 2002.

scale had ten points that radiated outwards like the spokes of a wheel for each indicator of the three growth areas. Each scale was joined together following an assessment by the village members to provide a visual representation of growth and development. However, the approach did not promote strategic planning and used a total of 18 complex, inter-related indicators such as equity and solidarity for village development, which are difficult to conceptualize.

In a similar approach Bjaras et al. (1991) developed a 'spider web' (so called due to its appearance being similar to a spider web) configuration for the measurement of community participation in Sweden. This approach has been used in evaluating community participation in other health programmes (Bopp et al., 1999; Hawe et al., 2000; Rifkin et al., 1988). Bjaras et al. used the approach for five factors to assess community participation: leadership, needs assessment, management, organization and resource mobilization; and a rating scale of narrow, medium and wide to rank each factor. The approach was not carried out as a self-assessment, however, but used an external agent; it did not promote strategic planning or self-improvement.

Figure 9.1 provides an example of a self-assessment of two women's groups in Nepal also using the spider web configuration to provide a visual representation of community empowerment (Gibbon et al., 2002) which, in this instance, the author referred to as 'community capacity'. This assessment used a ten-point rating scale. The numbers used to assess community capacity have little cross-comparison meaning. They only make sense relative to changes in the same scale by the same group or community over time or, as in this instance, similarities or differences between different stakeholders. The spider web was plotted out on newsprint by the co-worker and two women's groups, who found the information it provided helpful for comparing changes over time and important for discussing why they had given slightly different assessments for the same domain.

Graphing differences over time allows some conclusions to be drawn about community capacity/empowerment building. Differences between stakeholders at the same point in time, however, require facilitated discussion over why different ratings were assigned. For purposes of evaluating changes some consensus amongst stakeholders for ratings at any given time needs to be pursued.

In this chapter I have discussed how to plan and evaluate health promotion programmes so that they help to enhance community empowerment. In the next and final chapter I reflect back on the central theme of the book and discuss some of the social and political issues involved in advancing an empowering health promotion practice.

10 Implications for an Empowering Health Promotion Practice

In this final chapter I bring together the central themes of the book: power and empowerment, and discuss the broader implications of implementing these concepts to provide an empowering health promotion practice.

As I explain in Chapter 2, to promote health we must have clear strategies at all levels that work towards the elimination of poverty (reducing the gap between the rich and the poor) and the reduction of social inequalities (transforming unequal power relationships). Health, therefore, is a product of many different but closely related areas, for example, housing, transport, employment, community health services and social support. Health is also a product of a global market and strategies must increasingly cross national as well as organizational boundaries. What this means is that health promoters must work in collaboration with practitioners in many other sectors if they are to develop strategies to address poverty and social inequalities.

Health promoters cannot be expected to have an influence on health across all sectors and at all levels in their everyday work. However, there are two key areas of importance in which health promoters do have an influence:

- Health promoters are involved in influencing policies and practices that affect health, from national 'down' to the community level. In order to influence policy and practice, health promoters need to have a better understanding of the meaning of power and how the relationships between different stakeholders are understood and appropriately acted upon by the profession. This is explained in Chapter 3 (Power Transformation and Health Promotion Practice).
- Health promoters are involved in bottom-up or community development approaches in their day-to-day work that enable individuals and communities to have greater influence over the actions that can bring about social and political change. This is the process of 'community empowerment' and can lead to an influence on public policies, economic and regulatory changes through collective action, voting, lobbying political representatives and campaigning. To be effective in their work health promoters need to have a clear understanding about the influences on the process of community

empowerment. This is explained in Chapters 4 (Community Empowerment and Health Promotion Practice) and 7 (The Domains of Community Empowerment).

The reorientation of professional practice in health promotion towards power transformation and empowerment must be accompanied by a corresponding clarification of how these concepts can be practically accommodated within health promotion practice. This is explained in Chapters 5 (Addressing the Tensions in Health Promotion Programming) and 6 ('Parallel-tracking' Community Empowerment into Health Promotion Programming). The implementation of community empowerment in a programme context is explained in Chapter 8 (Building Community Empowerment Approaches in Health Promotion). The evaluation of community empowerment is explained in Chapter 9 (Evaluating Community Empowerment approaches).

However, innovations in practice must at the same time be accompanied by a redress of the constraints placed on health promotion by its bureaucratic nature and by the problematic relationship that exists between the state and civil society (defined here as people, in their capacity as citizens, associating with each other in social organizations such as clubs, religious groups, community betterment societies and public interest groups). The agencies that fund and implement health promotion must relinquish some of their power-over ('expert-dominance' and access to resources) in top-down programming to allow the elements of an empowering health promotion practice, discussed in this book, to become possible. Bottom-up programmes are dependent on funding and their continued support relies much on there being a political will to implement them. This may be difficult when the goal of the individuals and groups who are involved in community empowerment (civil society) is to bring about a change in the social and political order that challenges the very agencies (the state) that provide the funding for their continuation.

To explain this I examine three important external contexts that influence an empowering health promotion practice: political, economic and socio-cultural. I then examine the organizational context in which health promotion practitioners work and discuss how this can provide more scope and opportunity to embrace empowerment. I also discuss some of the limitations of using an empowering approach and the implications of these constraints to health promotion practice.

The influence of the political context

My introductory story about Rudolf Virchow in Chapter 1 argued that all diseases have political as well as pathological causes. Health promotion, and certainly its empowering form, is political, in so far as its actions depend on, and have some consequences for, the political context in which its practice occurs. The political context (defined here as those in governance with decision- and policy-making control) can be supportive or unsupportive towards community empowerment programmes. In either case the political context can act as a 'trigger' for individuals and groups to embark on the process of community empowerment.

If local communities are to participate in a meaningful way in bottom-up programmes there must be a political commitment to and resources for such participation at all governance levels. If a supportive political context does not exist the community must seize power through collective mobilization and action, first at a localized level and then through broader-scale social and political change.

To clarify these circumstances I distinguish between three 'scenarios' of community empowerment within differing political contexts (see Figure 10.1): a supportive political context; an uncooperative political context; and an unsupportive political context.

Scenario 1: A supportive political context

A supportive political context allows community empowerment approaches to develop under negotiated conditions in programmes with governmental and non-governmental organizations. People are assisted to gain power through the transformation of relationships, resource delivery and capacity building. Examples of this scenario have been used throughout the book (see Boxes 5.4, 7.3 and 7.5, on pages 70, 92 and 96 respectively). This is the scenario that Virchow (discussed in Chapter 1), in his life-long political commitment to health promotion, helped to create and that those of us living, and practising health promotion, in Western democracies still enjoy today.

Scenario 2: An uncooperative political context

This describes a context in which empowerment 'struggles' increasingly develop under conditions that do not readily allow negotiation with outside agencies and can involve strategies such as protests and lobbying. The political context, though seeking to minimize these disruptions, does not forcibly repress them. These actions can be seen in everyday life in many democratic and transitional economies, for example, the localized actions of residents in response to environmental threats or hazards (see Box 4.4 on page 56) or the wider actions of citizens demonstrating on the streets against undemocratic or corrupt governance in their country. Scenarios 1 and 2 describe the circumstances under which many health promoters presently work in a programme context.

This is also the scenario that Virchow was able to join after the initial street protests and labour movements in mid-nineteenth century Europe created a more democratic space in government.

Figure 10.1   The influence of the political context on community empowerment

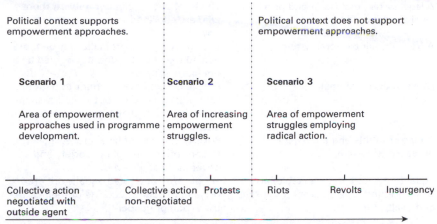

Political context supports empowerment approaches.		Political context does not support empowerment approaches.
Scenario 1	**Scenario 2**	**Scenario 3**
Area of empowerment approaches used in programme development.	Area of increasing empowerment struggles.	Area of empowerment struggles employing radical action.

Collective action negotiated with outside agent   Collective action non-negotiated   Protests   Riots   Revolts   Insurgency

Increasingly uncooperative political environments and a lack of government support for community empowerment

Source: Laverack, 1999: 173.

Scenario 3: An unsupportive political context

This describes a political context that does not support community involvement and may resist empowerment approaches. This is often accompanied by an increase in political instability and oppressive forms of governance and hegemonic power in civil society. Social justice and equity in society do not exist and this can lead to circumstances in which people can lose their basic rights to vote, protest or take legal action against those in authority (see Table 10.1).

Frances Piven and Richard Cloward (1977), two early writers on community organization, suggest that in conditions of extreme inequality and poverty, which are indicative of an unsupportive state or one dominated by élite group interests, poor people cannot maintain organizations or rely upon support from the established system. They must use the only significant resource they have: the capacity to cause trouble. The tactics used are protests, strikes, riots, revolts and insurgency. The disruption, public support and the reaction of the opposition become the basis for political influence. This is a limited option and only possible under extreme and specific circumstances such as extreme poverty, political instability and periods of social conflict. Piven and Cloward point out that historically this option has given rise to examples of dramatic social and political change resulting from collective (community) action such as the

Table 10.1   Basic rights and the political context

Supportive political context	Unsupportive political context
A legal system that is just and provides legal assistance for the poor.	The legal system is biased toward those who are educated and who already hold power.
A free and fair electoral system.	Voting is rigged, marginalized groups are denied the vote, the country is ruled by a one-party system.
Free expression of opinions.	People do not have the right to petition, to protest, to publish or to publicly speak their views that challenge those already in power.
An incorruptible and fair legal and bureaucratic system.	Poverty and lack of legal process give rise to corruption throughout society and governance at all levels.
Equal (or needs-based equitable) access to services including education, welfare and health care.	People are not treated equally but are prejudiced against because of their caste, tribe, clan or gender.

Source: Laverack, 1999: 144.

protests and riots amongst the lower-classes over rent increases in the US during the middle years of the twentieth century.

In such instances of radical community action, organizers (outside agents) and community groups need to maximize their efforts and push for full concessions in return for a cease to the disruptions. This can be a costly and risky strategy, but it is also the most effective means of utilizing the limited resources available to the very poor and marginalized.

Barbara Gray (1989), a seminal writer on inter-organizational collaboration and partnerships, comments that often 'weaker parties must first develop their capacity as stakeholders', usually through conflict and struggle, before the conditions for partnership – between the state and civil society – can exist. For example, most social movements begin by directly confronting social systems and stakeholders who hold power-over their members. The US civil rights movement used sit-ins and other forms of non-violent demonstration to physically prevent the apartheid exclusion of black people from neighbourhoods. The environment movement, to gain a seat in the corporate-government boardrooms where environmental policies were being formed, engaged in 'direct action' campaigns that blocked effluent pipes, stopped polluting activities or prevented whaling, logging or other forms of unsustainable resource extraction.

This is the scenario that Virchow encountered when his first indictment of the 'pathology' of early nineteenth century capitalism proved too challenging for powerful, and power-over, vested interests, prompting him to take action on the streets.

Ruth Sutherland (2002), a senior community development worker in Northern Ireland, identifies the key challenges that face health promoters in a country without peace and political stability: democracy and devolution. A political context that is stable and is not challenged by community empowerment and a community/voluntary sector that has the confidence and vision to adopt the role of enabling individuals to take collective action. Ruth Sutherland also identifies the political agenda, one that supports equality, and the ability and motivation of statutory organizations to provide the necessary support to bottom-up approaches, as important political challenges for the development of an empowering health promotion practice.

The influence of the economic context

The political and economic contexts are highly entwined. Politics defines who has authority; economics determines who has resources. Gill Gordon (1995) argues in her case study of sexual health in Africa that empowerment programmes cannot succeed unless people are supported by an economic context that provides basic resources such as incomes, food stuffs and shelter and is expanding to offer choices that present hope. For example, unemployment can lead to conflict, violence and crime in an effort by people to provide an income for themselves and their family. This can lead to feelings of vulnerability and powerlessness amongst individuals, groups and communities and can be the 'trigger' that begins the process of community empowerment.

Maruja Barrig (1990) provides an example of how the economic context did create the circumstances that were 'favourable' for community action. Women in Peru, forced by an economic crisis that led to depressed incomes and unemployment, decided to take action and empower themselves. Individual women working in community projects initially received government food aid. However, community organizations were quickly established by the women to run communal kitchens so as to more effectively channel relief to people in shanty towns. What was remarkable was the size and the permanence of these community organizations and the momentum that they created to lead the women on to further action. The economic context had created the desperate conditions that provided a 'trigger' for individual women to embark on the process of community empowerment.

Tackling health inequalities and narrowing the gap between the rich and the poor involves transforming unequal power relations by changing the economic context through long-term and practical strategies. For example, lowering unemployment, equal and fair pay and providing individuals with the skills necessary to fulfil their potential to work. Health promoters can have an influence in this through policy change and, perhaps more significantly, through enabling others, especially the marginalized and socially isolated, to have a greater level of participation in the political process.

However, community empowerment, which begins at a localized level and moves towards involving individuals into more broadly based actions, can become self-limiting. Individuals may become overwhelmed by the 'bigger picture' in which their smaller (localized) concerns exist and people may simply not be interested in engaging economic issues at the national or international levels. Two strategies that have proved to be relatively successful in Canada in addressing this limitation are:

- Ensuring public participation and the representation of community groups in governing or advisory boards and committees to health authorities to maintain pressure on addressing the underlying health determinants (Chapter 2).
- Building a broader base of community support for advocacy initiatives, for example, involving local groups and organizations in the decision-making processes in developing a campaign targeted at national level policy makers (Labonte, 1998).

There is a real risk that community empowerment approaches working to integrate the socially marginalized into the economic mainstream do not also challenge the economic mainstream as being inherently socially marginalizing. As Friedmann concludes in his important essay on empowerment strategies for alternative development in poorer countries:

> To be small and local is not enough… Political and economic empowerment, the inclusion of the excluded, is not generally part of a people-centred development approach. (1992: 158)

This is part of the now dominant economic discourse of 'neoliberalism', which emphasizes economic growth through free markets, minimal state regulation, privatization of state enterprises and minimal state welfare provision. It places an emphasis on competitiveness, individualism and meritocracy. This raises the question 'To what extent can empowerment occur in an economic context that is inherently based on status and hierarchy?' How, for example, can the principles of empowerment be applied in health promotion practice in a social and health system that regards workers' smoking habits to be a more important issue than the minimum wage or unemployment? (Carey, 2000). The discourse of neoliberalism has created economic pressures on governments to reduce taxation, labour regulations and social spending and prevents investment in sectors such as community empowerment that promote localized self-determination. Community empowerment must do more than simply integrating the marginalized by ensuring that there are explicit frameworks and 'tools' for the social and political analysis of power relationships, such as discussed in Chapters 2, 4 and 6 in this book.

The influence of the socio-cultural context

The socio-cultural context, expressed here as societal and cultural attitudes, beliefs, values and practices, can support community empowerment, for example, by creating an atmosphere in which interpersonal elements of social support on non-exclusive social networks can develop. Social capital (the features of social organization, networking, trust and collaboration) is an important element of the socio-cultural context and is discussed in Chapter 2.

The socio-cultural context can also be unsupportive towards community empowerment. In many parts of rural Asia traditional authority relations continue to dominate village life (Asthana, 1994). The socio-cultural tendency is for communities to follow strong leadership rather than make collective decisions. Such concentrated leadership offers limited scope for participation in decision-making and community empowerment. Local leaders do have the authority to mobilize community members to undertake development activities but often choose not to do so in order to maintain control within the community.

Marilyn Taylor (1995), a community development researcher and activist, discusses the socio-cultural changes that have taken place in South Africa since and during apartheid, and that have led to a rise in youth violence and criminal activity creating social conflict. Fear and violence are still part of everyday life that traumatizes individuals, families and communities (Taylor, 1995). The disintegration of the country's social fabric that resulted from the violence of apartheid has had a devastating effect on communities and created an atmosphere that has not facilitated empowerment. Fear and feelings of powerlessness within a society can create an apathy toward social justice. Pragmatically, I consider social justice to be the equitable access to resources and services allowing people to gain satisfaction on issues that influence their lives, without preventing other people from achieving similar satisfaction. Marilyn Taylor (1995) uses the term 'violence' to mean more than acts of aggression of one person against another and includes the institutionalized acts of oppression used by the apartheid system. These socio-cultural changes created tensions between youth, family and society, exacerbated by the breakdown of the education and welfare system. Subsequent development projects that placed an emphasis on narrowly defined economic growth measures further diminished support to many people and the potential for community empowerment.

An empowering approach to health promotion therefore requires, at the least, a moderately democratic political context, some economic resources and a culture that is moving towards non-coercive and non-patriarchal forms of leadership and organization. But it also requires funders, an organizational base and a professional orientation that both understands and has some commitment to support an empowering practice.

The influence of the organizational context

My argument in Chapter 1 was that health promotion is a bureaucratic activity carried out by or within governmental organizations or government-funded NGOs. These organizations operate at different levels between the state and civil society and between formal agencies and the community.

Various studies of governments and NGOs that have embraced health promotion's empowering discourse find that the concept of empowerment used in policy and in practice are often quite different, and, despite the intent to 'empower' communities, organizations and their staff tended to retain control over programming (Grace, 1991; Turbyne, 1996). Organizations remain chained to traditional ways of thinking and acting, ways that are bureaucratic and which inhibit the effective inclusion of empowering approaches.

But governments and bureaucracies, at least in democratic countries, are not monolithic entities. Not only are there often contradictions between the policies and actions of different government agencies, but also different civil servants and programme workers with differing ideas often exist and work together. There are opportunities of empowering potential within even the largest, most rigid bureaucracies. To take advantage of these opportunities the health promotion profession must address the philosophical nature, discourse and ideology, and the organizational context (the power relationships, structures and procedures) of agencies at all levels.

For there to be a philosophical shift in practice, health promoters could begin with a renaissance of the 'empowerment culture'. This advocates for participation and equity in health and was championed by the 'new health promotion movement' in the 1980s. These principles are still central to health promotion today and should not be lost because of the difficulties in making the concept of community empowerment operational. Health promoters should be encouraged to think, talk and write about health and the determinants of health in the context of both individual and collective empowerment. This must be reflected in the discourse of health promotion: the language, rhetoric, values and ideas and in the use of an emancipatory ideology that is conscious in linking the power relationships and processes between the individual and the political.

Health promotion, as defined in this book, is concerned with people and communities 'out there' in civil society. But empowerment must also occur within the profession of health promoters and in the organizations that employ them from the top tiers of policy and planning 'down' to the people working at the interface with the community. It is precisely this type of a fundamental issue that must be addressed if health promoters are to engage an empowering approach to practice. Health promotion agencies must build their organizational capacity and strengthen management practices, internal structures and the commitment to pursue empowerment approaches at all levels (international, state, NGO, and community organizations).

To achieve this, organizations should have a better understanding of the meaning of power and community empowerment (Chapters 3 and 4) and possess the practical 'tools' to enable communities to transform their identified needs and concerns into action. Community empowerment as a central theme of health promotion has existed for almost two decades but its practical application still remains elusive. Without the necessary 'tools' health promotion runs the risk of continuing to use the discourse of empowerment and participation because it allows them to be seen to involve the community but does not hold the responsibility of actively assisting people to seize or gain power towards social and political change.

Empowerment is usually theorized as a cross-sectoral and multi-faceted (individual, organizational and community) phenomenon and as such it should not be constrained by vertical programmes or sectorally specialist agencies. It cuts across programmes and the means to implement and measure empowerment approaches can be included as part of all sectors. The operational domains discussed in Chapter 7 have relevance to the work of many other sectors including education, primary health care and sustainable livelihoods, as communities organize and mobilize themselves towards social and political change. The process of 'parallel tracking' and the inclusion of empowerment goals have real potential as a part of the design of many types of health promotion programmes.

However, health promotion organizations are becoming increasingly tied to economic and quantifiable health targets as a consequence of national policies. This does not promote either innovation or the effectiveness of programmes and may restrict the range of health promotion activities, including bottom-up and empowering approaches. Health promotion programmes are increasingly expected to prove their cost effectiveness and this places demands for a higher level of skills and experience by programme managers. More sophisticated methods of evaluation can make health authorities less willing to transfer authority to less experienced community members in bottom-up approaches. The incentive of many funders to maintain power-over programming is now partly an attempt to ensure their own financial and political accountability. This makes empowerment, an especially difficult concept to implement and measure, an unattractive approach and raises the question 'How can dis-empowered (lack of funding, understanding and practical 'tools') health promoters facilitate community empowerment?' This book attempts to address this and other issues.

Power through health promotion

Can community power be gained through health promotion practice? In its present form dominated by top-down programming, bureaucratic systems and an undercurrent of authoritative power-over relationships and budget restrictions, it would seem unlikely. But this book, in the spirit of optimism that is to be found in much health promotion practice, has identified several ways in reaching closer towards the goal of more empowered communities.

We, as health promoters, need to recognize that working in empowering ways is very much a political activity and one that may have to use confrontation techniques to force the more powerful to negotiate terms with the less, but increasingly, empowered. Even within a programme context community empowerment approaches may require periods of disruptive political activity before the conditions for negotiation are possible. The structures of power-over, of bureaucracy and authority remain dominant in professional practice and part of the role of health promotion is to strive to challenge this situation.

In 1986 the Ottawa Charter for Health Promotion was written in the spirit of the social movements of the 1960s and 1970s and the thinking of community development and community organization activists such as Saul Alinsky and Paulo Freire. Whilst most health promoters would agree that the spirit of the Ottawa Charter is still as relevant today, they would also have to agree that the profession has failed to achieve the systematic empowerment of individuals, groups and communities.

This book has been written with the belief that the principles of community empowerment remain at the heart of health promotion practice and offers a fresh look at how we as practitioners can be more critical about whether our work is as empowering as it could be. However, there are two important issues that I feel should be considered by health promoters before embarking on a more empowering practice:

- There is another face to community empowerment, one that is viewed as being negative and associated with the use of force and violence to attain social and political change through intimidation, fear and coercion. It is a reflection that some people believe that it is better to be empowered than to be right.

  The interpretation of community empowerment as a process along a dynamic continuum shares the same elements for people involved in activities such as terrorism, as for example, residents acting against a waste dump or dog fouling in their community. The members of anti-social groups may hold idealistic views but they may also be highly motivated and share common beliefs and concerns. The members, who form cohesive groups and networks, make up a 'community' which in their view must bring about social and political change in their favour. How will society deal with such 'communities' once they have become empowered?

- At present there exists a contradiction between discourse and practice in health promotion: many health promoters continue to exert power-over the community through top-down programmes whilst at the same time using the emancipatory discourse of the Ottawa Charter. In this book I have argued that this contradiction continues because often: health promoters have a superficial understanding of the meaning of power and how the relationships between different stakeholders are understood and appropriately acted upon by the profession; and health promoters lack clarity about the influences on the process of community empowerment.

The danger of this contradiction is that it presents an illusion of choice and can act to hide an agenda of more typical top-down approaches, that is, coercing and manipulating people into doing what we want them to do, even against their will (power-over). Health promotion becomes a method of social and financial control, the very opposite of the spirit of the Ottawa Charter. Do health promoters want to help people or to change people?

And finally, the world has changed since the publication of the Ottawa Charter in 1986. If health promotion and its practitioners are to be empowering for the greater number of people in societies, especially the marginalized, they must now also support and contribute to building broad-based social coalitions concerned with issues such as globalization, fragmentation and the information revolution (Tudor-Smith and Farley, 1997). These coalitions are essential to create public policies that minimize, through redistribution and regulation, the disempowering effects of increasingly globalized, political and economic practices.

Chris Tudor-Smith and Peter Farley (1997), two senior health promoters involved in research, education and development in the UK, point out that the delivery of public services, industry and governance are fragmenting. This provides more diversification and specialization making it increasingly difficult to offer a holistic approach to promoting health. However, it also offers an opportunity to build community action to act upon common concerns of these fragmented groups and organizations. One opportunity will involve encouraging communities to gain better access to information through the fast growing number of resources such as the Internet. These resources can help to connect individuals and groups globally, to build networks and to share information and experiences to gain greater international support for issues of common concern.

Health promotion is now a global concern and collaboration for better health involves strategies that cross over different nations, international organizations and multi-national corporations; for example, a reduction in tobacco sales in one country can have serious economic, and hence health, implications in another country. Communities will need to be empowered to address their global concerns, first by making people aware of their own responsibilities and then by helping them to take the necessary actions to influence international policy.

This books presents the challenge to health promoters who wish to adopt an 'empowering practice' in their work: to find the ways to strengthen individuals' power-from-within and then to assist them to organize collectively to exercise their power-over the influences on their lives and health. The best summary that I have come across of what this presence means in practice is from an Australian Aboriginal organizer, Lily Walker, who is quoted as saying:

> If you are here to help me, then you are wasting your time. But if you come because your liberation is bound up in mine, then let us begin. (Valvarde, 1991)

The challenge lies in the role of the health promoter as a motivational and power-transforming (both for the health promoter and the 'community') presence and how this creates an empowering health promotion practice.

Bibliography

Abbott, J. (1995) 'Community participation and its relationship to Community Development', *Community Development Journal*, 30 (2): 158–68.

Adams, L., Amos, M. and Munro, J. (eds) (2002) *Promoting health: Politics and practice*. London: Sage.

Adams, R.N. (1977) 'Power in human societies: a synthesis', in R.D. Fogelson and R.N. Adams (eds), *The anthropology of power: ethnographic studies from Asia, Oceania, and the New World*. New York: Academic Press. pp. 387–410.

Aggleton, P. (1991) *Health*. London: Routledge.

Ahuja, K. (1994) 'Mobilization of rural women through voluntary efforts – a case study', *Studies in Third World Societies*, 51 (March): 1–10.

Airhihenbuwa, C.O. (1994) 'Health Promotion and the Discourse on Culture: Implications for Empowerment', Health Education Quarterly, 21 (3): 345–53.

Albert, J. (1992) 'If we don't do it, it won't get done: a case study from Nicaragua', *International Social Work*, 35 (2): 229–41.

Alinsky, S.D. (1969) *Reveille for Radicals*. New York: Vintage Books.

Alinsky, S.D. (1972) *Rules For Radicals: A practical primer for realistic radicals*. New York: Vintage Books.

Arnstein, S.R. (1969) 'A Ladder of Citizen Participation', *Journal of the American Institute of Planners*, July: 216–23.

Asthana, S. (1994) 'Community participation in health and development' in D. Phillips and Y. Verhasselt (eds), *Health and Development*. London: Routledge. pp. 182–96.

Auslander, G. (1988) 'Social Networks and the Functional Health Status of the Poor: A Secondary Analysis of Data from the National Survey of Personal Health Practices and Consequences', *Journal of Community Health*, 13 (4).

Baistow, K. (1995) 'Liberation and regulation? Some paradoxes of empowerment', *Critical Social Policy*, (42): 34–46.

Bakhteari, Q.A. (1988) 'Building on Traditional Patterns for Women Empowerment at Grassroots Level', *Development*, (4): 55–60.

Barr, A. (1995) 'Empowering communities – beyond fashionable rhetoric? Some reflections on Scottish experience', *Community Development Journal*, 30 (2): 121–32.

Barrig, M. (1990) 'Women and Development in Peru: Old Models, New Actors', *Community Development Journal*, 25 (4): 377–85.

Baum, F. (1990) 'The new public health: force for change or reaction?', *Health Promotion International*, 5 (2): 145–50.

Baum, F. (1995) 'Researching Public Health: Behind the Qualitative–Quantitative Methodological Debate', *Social Science Medicine*, 40 (4): 459–68.

Bell, C. and Newby, H. (1978) *Community Studies*. London: George Allen and Unwin.

Bell-Woodard, G. (2002) 'The development of a community active living initiative: Saskatoon in motion', Community Alliances for Health Research (CAHR) in motion. University of Saskatoon, Saskatoon, Canada.

Berger, P. and Neuhaus, R. (1977) To empower people: The role of mediating structures in public policy. Studies in political and social processes. Washington: American Enterprise Institute for Public Policy Research.

Berkeley, N., Goodall, G., Noon, D. and Collis, C. (1995) 'Involving the community in plan preparation', Community Development Journal, 30 (2): 189–99.

Berkman, L. (1986) 'Social networks, support and health: taking the next step forward', American Journal of Epidemiology, 123 (4): 559–61.

Bernstein, E., Wallerstein, N., Braithwaite, R., Gutierrez, L., Labonte, R. and Zimmerman, M. (1994) 'Empowerment forum: a dialogue between guest editorial board members', Health Education Quarterly, 21 (3): 281–94.

Bjaras, G., Haglund, B.J.A. and Rifkin, S.B. (1991) 'A new approach to community participation assessment', Health Promotion International, 6 (3): 199–206.

Blaxter, M. (1990) Health and Lifestyles. New York: Routledge.

Bloor, M. and McIntosh, J. (1990) 'Surveillance and concealment', in S. Cunningham-Burley and N.P. McKeganey (eds), Readings in Medical Sociology. New York: Tavistock/Routledge.

Bopp, M., Germann, K., Bopp, J., Littlejohns, L.B. and Smith, N. (1999) Assessing Community Capacity for Change. Calgary: Four Worlds Development.

Boutilier, M. (1993) 'The Effectiveness of Community Action in Health Promotion: A Research Perspective'. Toronto: University of Toronto. ParticiACTION. 3.

Bracht, N. and Tsouros, A. (1990) 'Principles and strategies of effective community participation', Health Promotion International, 5 (3): 199–208.

Braddy, B.A., Orenstein, D., Brownstein, J.N. and Cook, T.J. (1992) 'PATCH: An Example of Community Empowerment for Health', Journal of Health Education, 23 (3): 179–82.

Braithwaite, R.L., Bianchi, C. and Taylor, S.E. (1994) 'Ethnographic Approach to Community Organisation and Health Empowerment', Health Empowerment, 21 (3): 407–16.

Britten, N. (1995) 'Qualitative interviews in medical research', British Medical Journal, 311 (July): 251–3.

Brown, D. (1991) 'Methodological considerations in the evaluation of social development programmes – an alternative approach', Community Development Journal, 26 (4): 259–65.

Bryman, A. (1992) Quantity and Quality in Social Research. London: Routledge.

Burgess, R.G. (1982) Field Research: A source book and field manual. London: Allen and Unwin.

Burgess, R.G. (1984) In the Field: An introduction to field research. London: George Allen and Unwin.

Butterfoss, F.D., Goodman, R.M. and Wandersman, A. (1996) 'Community Coalitions for Prevention and Health Promotion: Factors Predicting Satisfaction, Participation and Planning', Health Education Quarterly, 23 (1): 65–79.

Canadian Public Health Association (1996) 'Action Statement for Health Promotion in Canada', available at http://www.cpha.ca. 29.05.98.

Carey, P. (2000) 'Community health and empowerment', in J. Kerr (ed.), Community Health Promotion: Challenges for practice. London: Bailliere Tindall.

Christian, J. (1993) 'Community: An Indian perspective', Together (July-September): 6–7.

CIDA (1996) *A Project Level Handbook: The why and how of Gender Sensitive Indicators*. Hull, Quebec: CIDA.

Clark, J. (1991) *Democratizing Development: The role of voluntary organizations*. West Hartford: Kumarian Press.

Clark, N.M., Baker, E.A., Chawla, A. and Maru, M. (1993) 'Sustaining collaborative problem solving: strategies from a study in six Asian countries', *Health Education Research. Theory and Practice*, 8 (3): 385–402.

Cohen, D.R. and Henderson, J.B. (1991) *Health, Prevention and Economics*. Oxford: Oxford University Press.

Cohen, J. (1985) 'Strategy or identity: new theoretical paradigms and contemporary social movements', *Social research*, 52 (4): 663–716.

Cohen, S. and Syme, L. (eds) (1985) *Social Support and Health*. Toronto: Academic Press.

Conger, J. and Kanungo, R. (1988) 'The Empowerment Process: Integrating Theory and Practice', *Academy of Management Review*, 13 (3): 471–82.

Constantino-David, K. (1995) 'Community Organising in the Philippines: The Experience of Development NGOs', in G. Craig and M. Mayo (eds), *A Reader in Participation and Development*. London: Zed Books. pp. 154–67.

Cooke, B. and Kothari, U. (eds) (2001) *The Case for Participation as Tyranny*. London: Zed Books.

Cracknell, B.E. (1996) 'Evaluating Development Aid', *Evaluation*, 2 (1): 23–33.

Craig, G. and Mayo, M. (eds) (1995) *Community Empowerment: A Reader in Participation and Development*. London: Zed Books.

Dahlgren, G. and Whitehead, M. (1992) *Policies and Strategies to Promote Equity in Health*. Copenhagen: World Health Organization Regional Office for Europe.

Dines, A. and Cribb, A. (eds) (1993) *Health Promotion: Concepts and practice*. Oxford: Blackwell Science.

Downie, R.S., Tannahill, C. and Tannahill, A. (1996) *Health Promotion: Models and values, 2nd edn*. Oxford: Oxford University Press.

Duignan, P., Casswell, S., Chapman, P., Barnes, H., Allan, B. and Conway, K. (2001) *Background Report on the Draft Project Indicators Framework*. Wellington, New Zealand: Public Health Policy Group.

Durning, A.B. (1989) 'Action at the grassroots: Fighting poverty and environmental decline', *Worldwatch*, 2 (6): 88.

Ehrenreich, J. (ed.) (1978) *The Cultural Crisis of Modern Medicine*. New York: Monthly Review Press.

Eisen, A. (1994) 'Survey of neighbourhood-based, comprehensive community empowerment initiatives', *Health Education Quarterly*, 21 (2): 235–52.

Eng, E. and Parker, E. (1994) 'Measuring community competence in the Mississippi Delta: the interface between programme evaluation and empowerment', *Health Education Quarterly*, 21 (2): 199–220.

Eng, E., Salmon, M.E. and Mullan, F. (1992) 'Community empowerment: the critical base for primary health care', *Family Community Health*, 15 (1): 1–12.

Erzinger, S. (1994) 'Empowerment in Spanish: words can get in the way', *Health Education Quarterly*, 21 (3): 417–19.

Evans, R., Barer, M. and Marmor, T. (eds) (1994) *Why Are Some People Healthy and Others Not? The Determinants of the Health of Populations*. New York: Aldine de Gruyter.

Evans, R.D. and Stoddart, G.L. (1990) 'Producing health, consuming health care', *Social Science and Medicine*, 31 (12): 1347–63.

Everson, S.A., Lynch, J.W., Chesney, M.A., Kaplan, G.A., Goldberg, D.E., Shade, S.B., Cohen, R.D., Salonen, R. and Salonen, J.T. (1997) 'Interaction of workplace demands and cardiovascular reactivity in progression of carotid atherosclerosis: population based study', *British Medical Journal*, 314: 553–8.

Ewles, L. and Simnett, I. (1999) *Promoting Health: A practical guide, 4th edn*. London: Bailliere Tindall.

Eyerman, R. and Jamison, A. (1991) *Social Movements: A cognitive approach*. Cambridge: Polity Press.

Fahlberg, L.L., Poulin, A.L., Girdano, D.A. and Dusek, D.E. (1991) 'Empowerment as an Emerging Approach in Health Education', *Journal of Health Education*, 22 (3): 185–93.

Farrant, W. (1991) 'Addressing the Contradictions. Health Promotion and Community Health in Action in the UK', *International Journal of Health Services*, 21 (3): 423–39.

Fawcett, S.B., Paine-Andrews, A., Francisco, V.T., Schultz, J.A., Richter, K.P., Lewis, R.K., Williams, E.L., Harris, K.J., Berkley, J.Y., Fisher, J.L. and Lopez, C.M. (1995) 'Using empowerment theory in collaborative partnerships for community health and development', *American Journal of Community Psychology*, 23 (5): 677–97.

Feather, J. and Labonte, R. (1995) *Sharing Knowledge from Health Promotion Practice*. Saskatoon: University of Saskatchewan, Praire Region Health Promotion Research Centre.

Fetterman, D.M., Kaftarian, S.J. and Wandersman, A. (eds) (1996) *Empowerment Evaluation: Knowledge and Tools for Self-Assessment and Accountability*. Thousand Oaks, CA: Sage.

Finsterbusch, K., Ingersoll, J. and Llewellyn, L. (1990) 'Methods for social analysis in developing countries', *Social Impact Assessment Series No. 17*. Boulder, CO: Westview Press.

Fisher, S.L. (ed.) (1993) *Fighting Back in Appalachia: Traditions of resistance and change*. Philadelphia, PA: Temple University Press.

Flick, L.H., Reese, C.G., Rogers, G., Fletcher, P. and Sonn, J. (1994) 'Building community for health: lessons from a seven-year-old neighborhood/university partnership', *Health Education Quarterly*, 21 (3): 369–80.

Flynn, B.C., Ray, D.W. and Rider, M.S. (1994) 'Empowering communities: action research through healthy cities', *Health Education Quarterly*, 21 (3): 395–405.

Foucault, M. (1979) *Discipline and Punishment: The birth of the prison*. London: Peregrine books.

Francisco, V.T., Paine, A.L. and Fawcett, S.B. (1993) 'A methodology for monitoring and evaluating community health coalitions', *Health Education Research. Theory and Practice*, 8 (3): 403–416.

Freire, P. (1973) *Education for Critical Consciousness*. New York: Seabury Press.

Freudenburg, N. (1997) *Health Promotion in the City*. Atlanta, GA: Centres for Disease Control and Prevention.

Friedmann, J. (1992) *Empowerment: the politics of alternative development*. Oxford: Blackwell.

Gajanayake, S. and Gajanayake, J. (1993) *Community Empowerment: A participatory training manual on community project development*. New York: PACT Publications.

Geyer, S. (1997) 'Some conceptual considerations on the sense of coherence', *Social Science Medicine*, 44 (12): 1771–9.

Gibbon, M. (1999) 'Meetings with meaning: health dynamics in rural Nepal', unpublished PhD thesis, South Bank University, London.

Gibbon, M., Labonte, R. and Laverack, G. (2002) 'Evaluating Community Capacity', *Health and Social Care in the Community*, 10 (6): 485–91.

Giddens, A. (1984) *The Constitution of Society*, Berkeley, CA: University of California Press.

Githumbi, S. (1993) 'Community: An African perspective', *Together*, (July-September): 6–7.

Glanz, K., Marcus-Lewis, F. and Rimer, B. (1990) *Health Behaviour and Health Education: Theory, research and practice*. Oxford: Jossey-Bass.

Goodman, R.M., Speers, M.A., McLeroy, K., Fawcett, S., Kegler, M., Parker, E., Rathgeb Smith, S., Sterling, T.D. and Wallerstein, N. (1998) 'Identifying and defining the dimensions of community capacity to provide a basis for measurement', *Health Education and Behavior*, 25 (3): 258–78.

Gordon, G. (1995) 'Participation, Empowerment and Sexual Health in Africa', in G. Craig and M. Mayo (eds), (1995) *Community Empowerment: A Reader in Participation and Development*. London: Zed Books. pp. 181–93.

Grace, V.M. (1991) 'The marketing of empowerment and the construction of the health consumer: a critique of health promotion', *International Journal of Health Services*, 21 (2): 329–43.

Gray, B. (1989) *Collaborating: Finding common ground for multiparty problems*. San Francisco, CA: Jossey-Bass.

Green, A. and Matthias, A. (1996) 'How should governments view nongovernmental organizations?', *World Health Forum*, 17: 42–5.

Green, L. and Kreuter, M. (1991) *Health Promotion Planning. An educational and environmental approach*. Toronto: Mayfield.

Green, L.W., George, M.A., Daniel, M., Frankish, C.J., Herbert, C.J., Bowie, W.R. and O'Neill, M. (1995) *Study of Participatory Research in Health Promotion*. Vancouver: Royal Society of Canada.

Gruber, J. and Trickett, E.J. (1987) 'Can we empower others? The paradox of empowerment in the governing of an alternative public school', *American Journal of Community Psychology*, 15 (3): 353–72.

Guzzo, R.A., Yost, P.R., Campbell, R.J. and Shea, G.P. (1993) 'Potency in groups: Articulating a construct', *British Journal of Social Psychology*, 32: 87–106.

Hancock, T., Labonte, R. and Edwards, R. (1999) 'Indicators that count: Measuring population health at the community level', *Canadian Journal of Public Health*, S22–S26.

Hatfield, A. (1998) 'Working together to reduce suicide in the farming community in North Yorkshire', in A. Scriven (ed.) *Alliances in Health Promotion: Theory and practice*. London: MacMillan pp. 132–42.

Hawe, P. (1994) 'Capturing the meaning of 'community' in community intervention evaluation. Some contributions from community psychology', *Health Promotion International*, 9 (3): 199–210.

Hawe, P., King, L., Noort, M., Jordens, C. and Lloyd, B. (2000) *Indicators to Help with Capacity Building in Health Promotion*. Sydney: Australian Centre for Health Promotion/NSW Health.

Hayes, B.E. (1994) 'How to Measure Empowerment', *Quality Progress*, February: 41–6.

Haynes, A.W. and Singh, R.N. (1993) 'Helping families in developing countries: A model based on family empowerment and social justice', *Social Development Issues*, 15 (1): 27–37.

Hildebrandt, E. (1996) 'Building community participation in health care: a model and example from South Africa', *Image: Journal of Nursing Scholarship*, 28 (2): 155–9.

Hindess, B. (1996) *Discourses of Power: From Hobbes to Foucault*. Oxford: Blackwell.

Hope, A. and Timmel, S. (1988) 'Training for Transformation', *Contact*, 106 (December): 4–7.

Huberman, A.M. and Miles, M.B. (1994) 'Data Management and Analysis Methods', in N.K. Denzin and Y.S. Lincoln (eds), *Handbook of Qualitative Research*. Thousand Oaks, CA: Sage pp. 428–44.

Hyndman, B. (1998) *Health Promotion Action: What works? What needs to be changed?*. Toronto: Centre for Health Promotion.

IRED (1997) *People's Empowerment. Grassroots Experiences in Africa, Asia and Latin America*. Rome: IRED-NORD.

Israel, B.A. (1985)'Social networks and social support: implications for natural helper and community level interventions', *Health Education Quarterly*, 12 (1): 65–80.

Israel, B.A., Checkoway, B., Schultz, A. and Zimmerman, M. (1994) 'Health education and community empowerment: conceptualizing and measuring perceptions of individual, organizational and community control', *Health Education Quarterly*, 21 (2): 149–70.

Israel, B.A., Cummings, K.M., Dignan, M.B., Heaney, C.A., Perales, D.P., Simons-Morton, B.G. and Zimmerman, M.A. (1995) 'Evaluation of health education programs: current assessment and future directions', *Health Education Quarterly*, 22 (3): 364–89.

Jackson, T., Mitchell, S. and Wright, M. (1989) 'The community development continuum', *Community Health Studies*, 8 (1): 66–73.

Jayaweera, S. (1997) 'Women, education and empowerment in Asia', *Gender and Education*, 9 (4): 411–23.

Jeffery, B. (2001) 'First Nation's Health Development: Tools for assessment of health and social service program impacts on community wellness and capacity'. Saskatoon: University of Regina.

Jones, A. (2002) 'Sustainable Livelihoods for Livestock Producing Communities in the Kyrgyz Republic'. Progress report, SLLPC, Bishkek, Kyrgyz, Republic.

Jones, L. and Sidell, M. (eds) (1997) *The Challenge of Promoting Health: Exploration and action*. London: MacMillan.

Jorgensen, D.L. (1989) *Participant Observation: A methodology for human studies*. London: Sage.

Kalyalya, D. (ed.) (1988) *Aid and Development in Southern Africa*. Atlantic City, NJ: Africa World Press.

Katz, R. (1984) 'Empowerment and Synergy: Expanding the Community's Healing Resources', in J. Rappaport (eds), *Studies in Empowerment: Steps toward understanding and action*. New York: Haworth Press. pp. 201–226.

Kawachi, I., Kennedy, B.P., Lochner, K. and Prothrow-Stith, D. (1997) 'Social capital, income equality and mortality', *American Journal of Public Health*, 87 (9): 1491–8.

Kegler, M.C., Steckler, A., Herndon Malek, S. and McLeroy, K. (1998) 'A multiple case study of implementation in 10 local project ASSIST coalitions in North Carolina', *Health Education Research. Theory and Practice*, 13 (2): 225–38.

Kelly, K. and Van Vlaenderen, H. (1996) 'Dynamics of Participation in a Community Health Project', *Social Science Medicine*, 24 (9): 1235–46.

Kieffer, C.H. (1984) 'Citizen Empowerment: A Development Perspective', *Prevention in Human Services*, 3: 9–36.

Kilian, A. (1988) 'Conscientisation: an empowering, nonformal education approach for community health workers', *Community Health Journal*, 23 (2): 117–23.

Kitzinger, J. (1995) 'Introducing focus groups', *British Medical Journal*, 311: 299–302.

Knox, C. and Hughes, J. (1994) 'Policy Evaluation in Community Development: Some Methodological Considerations', *Community Development Journal*, 29 (3): 239–50.

Korsching, P.F. and Borich, T.O. (1997) 'Facilitating cluster communities: lessons from the Iowa experience', *Community Development Journal*, 32 (4): 342–53.

Kretzmann, J. and McKnight, J. (1993) *Building Communities from the Inside Out*. Evanston, IL: Northwestern University Press.

Kroeker, C. (1995) 'Individual, organizational and societal empowerment: a study of the processes in a Nicaraguan agricultural cooperative', *American Journal of Community Psychology*, 23 (5): 749–64.

Kroutil, L.A. and Eng, E. (1989) 'Conceptualising and assessing potential for community participation: a planning method', *Health Education Research. Theory and Practice*, 4 (3): 305–19.

Kumpfer, K., Turner, C., Hopkins, R. and Librett, J. (1993) 'Leadership and team effectiveness in community coalitions for the prevention of alcohol and other drug abuse', *Health Education Research. Theory and Practice*, 8 (3): 359–74.

Labonte, R. (1989) 'Healthy public policy: a survey of Ontario health professionals', *International Quarterly of Community Health Education*, 9 (4): 321–42.

Labonte, R. (1990) 'Empowerment: Notes on Professional and Community Dimensions', *Canadian Review of Social Policy*, (26): 64–75.

Labonte, R. (1992) 'Heart health inequalities in Canada: Models, theory and planning', *Health Promotion International*, 7 (2): 119–28.

Labonte, R. (1993) *Health Promotion and Empowerment: Practice Frameworks*. Toronto: University of Toronto. ParticipACTION. 3.

Labonte, R. (1994) 'Health Promotion and Empowerment: Reflections on Professional Practice', *Health Education Quarterly*, 21 (2): 253–68.

Labonte, R. (1996) *Community Development in the Public Health Sector: The Possibilities of an Empowering Relationship Between the State and Civil Society*. Toronto: York University. PhD.

Labonte, R. (1998) *A Community Development Approach to Health Promotion: A background paper on practice tensions, strategic models and accountability requirements for health authority work on the broad determinants of health*. Edinburgh: Health Education Board for Scotland.

Labonte, R., Bell-Woodard, G., Chad, K. and Laverack, G. (2002) 'Community capacity building: From means to program end, to end from program means', *Canadian Journal of Public Health*, 93 (3): 181–2.

Labonte, R. and Edwards, R. (1995) *Equity in Action: Supporting the Public in Public Policy*. Toronto: Centre for Health Promotion/Participaction.

Labonte, R. and Robertson, A. (1996) 'Delivering the goods, showing our stuff: the case for a constructivist paradigm for health promotion and research', *Health Education Quarterly*, 23 (4): 431–47.

Lalonde, M. (1974) *A New Perspective on the Health of Canadians*. Ottawa: Department of Health and Welfare Canada.

Laverack, G. (1998) 'The concept of empowerment in a traditional Fijian context', *Journal of Community Health and Clinical Medicine for the Pacific*, 5 (1): 26–9.

Laverack, G. (1999) 'Addressing the contradiction between discourse and practice in health promotion', unpublished PhD thesis, Deakin University, Melbourne.

Laverack, G. (2001) 'An identification and interpretation of the organizational aspects of community empowerment', *Community Development Journal*, 36 (2): 40–52.

Laverack, G. (2003) 'Building Capable Communities: Experiences in a rural Fijian context', *Health Promotion International*, 18 (2): 99–106.

Laverack, G. and Labonte, R. (2000) 'A planning framework for the accommodation of community empowerment goals within health promotion programming', *Health Policy and Planning*, 15 (3): 255–62.

Laverack, G. and Wallerstein, N. (2001) 'Measuring community empowerment: a fresh look at organizational domains', *Health Promotional International*, 16 (2): 179–85.

Leach, F. (1994) 'Expatriates as Agents of Cross-Cultural Transmission', *Compare*, 24 (3): 217–31.

Leonard, B. and Leonard, S. (1991) *DUVATA: Management and planning in Fiji. The Ministry of Fijian Affairs*. Suva: Hanns Seidel Foundation.

Lerner, M. (1986) *Surplus Powerlessness*. Oakland, CA: The Institute for Labour and Mental Health.

LeVeen, D. (1983) 'Organisation or Disruption? Strategic options for marginal groups: The case of the Chicago Indian village', in Freeman, J. (ed.), *Social Movements of the Sixties and Seventies*. New York: Longman. pp. 211–34.

Lindbladh, E. and Hanson, B.S. (1993) 'A critical analysis of different leadership approaches to community health work in Kirseberg, Sweden', *Health Promotion International*, 8 (4): 291–7.

Linden, K. (1994) 'Health and Empowerment', *The Journal of Applied Social Sciences*, 18 (1): 33–40.

MaCallan, L. and Narayan, V. (1994) 'Keeping the heart beat in Grampian – a case study in community participation and ownership', *Health Promotion International*, 9 (1): 13–19.

Macdonald, G., Veen, C. and Tones, K. (1996) 'Evidence for success in health promotion: suggestions for improvement', *Health Education Research. Theory and Practice*, 11 (3): 367–76.

Macleod, M., Graham, G., Johnston, M., Dibben, C. and Briscoe, S. (1999) 'A comparison a day keeps the doctor away ... or does it?, *Health Variations*, (5): 10–11.

Mailbach, E. and Murphy, D.A. (1995) 'Self-efficacy in health promotion research and practice: conceptualization and measurement', *Health Education Research. Theory and Practice*, 10 (1): 37–50.

Marsden, D., Oakley, P. and Pratt, B. (1994) *Measuring the Process: Guidelines for evaluating social development*. Oxford: INTRAC.

Martin, M. (1994) 'Power and difference in participatory research: A reflection on process', in K. de Koorie (ed.), *The proceedings of an international symposium of participatory research in health promotion*. Liverpool: Liverpool School of Tropical Medicine. pp. 116–119.

Maton, K. and Salem, D. (1995) 'Organizational characteristics of empowering community settings: a multiple case study approach', *American Journal of Community Psychology*, 23 (5): 631–56.

McCall, M. (1988) 'The implications of Eastern African rural social structure for local level development: the case for participatory development based on indigenous knowledge systems', *Regional Development Dialogue*, 9 (2): 41–69.

McDonald, D.E. (1997) *Developing Guidelines to Enhance the Evaluation of Overseas Development Projects*. Melbourne: Overseas Service Bureau.

McFarlane, J. and Fehir, J. (1994) '*De Madres a Madres*. A community primary health care programme based on empowerment', *Health Education Quarterly*, 21 (3): 382–94.

McGraw, S.A., Stone, E.J., Osganian, S.K., Elder, J.P., Perry, C.L., Johnson, C.C., Parcel, G.S., Webber, L.S. and Luepker, R.V. (1994) 'Design of process evaluation within the child and adolescent trial for cardiovascular health (CATCH)', *Health Education Quarterly*, Supplement 2 (S5– S26).

McIntyre, S. (1986) 'The patterning of health by social position in contemporary Britain: directions for sociological research', *Social Science and Medicine*, 23 (4): 393–415.

McKnight, J.L. (1987) 'Regenerating community', *Social Policy*, 17 (3): 54–8.

McMillan, B., Florin, P., Stevenson, J., Kerman, B. and Mitchell, R.E. (1995) 'Empowerment praxis in community coalitions', *American Journal of Community Psychology*, 23 (5): 699–727.

Melucci, A. (1989) *Nomads of the Present: Social Movements and Individual Needs in Contemporary Society*. Philadelphia, PA: Temple University Press.

Minkler, M. (1985) 'Social support and the elderly', in S. Cohen and L. Syme (eds), *Social Support and Health*. Toronto: Academic Press.

Minkler, M. (1989) 'Health education, health promotion and the open society: an historical perspective', *Health Education Quarterly*, 16 (1): 17–30.

Minkler, M. (ed.) (1997) *Community Organizing and Community Building for Health*. New Brunswick: Rutgers University Press.

Minkler, M. and Cox, K. (1980) 'Creating critical consciousness in health: applications of Freire's philosophy and methods to the health care setting', *International Journal of Health Services*, 10 (2): 311–22.

Morriss, P. (1987) *Power: A philosophical analysis*. New York: St. Martin's Press.

Murray, S.A. and Graham, L.J.C. (1995) 'Practice-based needs assessment: use of four methods in a small neighbourhood', *British Medical Journal*, 310: 1443–8.

Neighbors, H., Braithwaite, R. and Thompson, E. (1995) 'Health promotion and African-Americans: from personal empowerment to community action', *American Journal of Health Promotion*, March/April (4): 281–7.

North York Community Health Promotion Research Unit (NYCHPRU)(1993), *Community Health Responses to Health Inequalities*. Toronto: NYCHPRU.

Nutbeam, D. (1997) *Health Promotion Glossary*. Geneva: World Health Organisation.

O'Connor, M.L. and Parker, E. (1995) *Health Promotion: Principles and practice in the Australian context*. Marrickville, NSW: Allen and Unwin.

O'Gorman, F. (1995) 'Brazilian Community Development: Changes and Challenges', in G. Craig and M. Mayo (eds), *Community Empowerment: A Reader in Participation and Development*. London: Zed Books. pp. 206–17.

O'Neill, M. (1992) 'Community participation in Quebec's health system: A strategy to curtail community empowerment', *International Journal of Health Services*, 22 (2): 287–301.

Oakley, P. (1991) *Projects with People: The practice of participation in rural development*. Geneva: International Labour Office.

Offe, C. (1984) *Contradictions of the Welfare State*. Boston, MA: MIT Press.

Olsen, M.E. and Marger, M.N. (eds) (1993) *Power in Modern Societies*. San Francisco, CA: Westview Press.

Ovrebo, B., Ryan, M., Jackson, K. and Hutchinson, K. (1994) 'The homeless prenatal program: a model for empowering homeless pregnant women', *Health Education Quarterly*, 21 (2): 187–98.

Pakulski, J. (1991) *Social Movements. The politics of moral protest*. Sydney: Longman Cheshire.

Palmer, C.T. and Anderson, M.J. (1986) 'Assessing the development of community involvement', *World Health Statistics Quarterly*, 39: 345–52.

Panet-Raymond, J. (1992) 'Partnership: Myth or reality?', *Community Development Journal*, 27 (2): 156–65.

Parsons, T. (1960) *Structure and Process in Modern Societies*. New York: Collier-MacMillan.

Patton, M.Q. (1997) 'Toward distinguishing empowerment evaluation and placing it in a larger context', *Evaluation Practice*, 18 (2): 147–63.

Pederson, A., O'Neill, M. and Rootman, I. (eds) (1994) *Health Promotion in Canada: Provincial, National and International Perspectives*. Toronto: W.B. Saunders.

Pelletier, D. and Jonsson, V. (1994) 'The use of information in the Iringa Nutrition Programme', *Food Policy*, 19 (3): 301–313.

Petersen, A.R. (1994) 'Community development in Health Promotion: empowerment or regulation?', *Australian Journal of Public Health*, 1 (2): 213–17.

Phillips, D.R. and Verhasselt, Y. (1994) *Health and Development*. New York: Routledge.

Piven, F.F. and Cloward, R. (1977) *Poor Peoples' Movements: Why they succeed, how they fail*. New York: Pantheon Books.

Plough, A. and Olafson, F. (1994) 'Implementing the Boston Healthy Start Initiative: a case study of community empowerment and public health', *Health Education Quarterly*, 21 (2): 221–34.

Poland, B., Green, L. and Rootman, I. (eds) (2000) *Settings for Health Promotion: linking theory and practice*. Newbury Park, CA: Sage.

Purdey, A.F., Adhikari, G.B., Robinson, S.A. and Cox, P.W. (1994) 'Participatory health development in rural Nepal: clarifying the process of community empowerment', *Health Education Quarterly*, 21 (3): 329–43.

Puska, P., Tuomilehto, J., Nissinen, A. and Vartiainen, E. (eds) (1995) *The North Karelia Project: 20 year results and experiences*. Helsinki: The National Public Health Institute.

Putnam, R.D., Leonardi, R. and Nanetti, R.Y. (1993) *Making Democracy Work: Civic Traditions in Modern Italy*. Princeton, NJ: Princeton University Press.

Raeburn, J. (1993) *How Effective is Strengthening Community Action as a Strategy for Health Promotion?* Toronto: University of Toronto. ParticiACTION. 3.

Raeburn, J. and Rootman, I. (1998) *People-Centred Health Promotion*. Chichester: John Wiley.

Rappaport, J. (1984) *Studies in Empowerment: Steps toward understanding and action*. New York: Haworth Press.

Rappaport, J. (1985) 'The Power of Empowerment Language', *Social Policy*, Fall: 15–21.

Rappaport, J. (1987) 'Terms of empowerment/exemplars of prevention. Toward a theory of community psychology', *American Journal of Community Psychology*, 15 (2): 121–47.

Raymond, J.S. and Patrick, W. (1988) 'Empowerment for primary health care and child survival. Escalating community participation, community competence and self reliance in the Pacific', *Asian Pacific Journal of Public Health*, 2 (2): 90–95.

Rebien, C.C. (1996) 'Participatory evaluation of development assistance. Dealing with power and facilitative learning', *Evaluation*, 2 (2): 151–71.

Reinelt, C. (1994) 'Fostering empowerment, building community: the challenge for state funded feminist organisations', *Human Relations*, 47 (6): 685–704.

Rifkin, S. (1995) 'Paradigms lost: toward a new understanding of community participation in health programmes', *Acta Tropica*, 61: 72–92.

Rifkin, S.B. (1990) *Community Participation in Maternal and Child Health/Family Planning Programmes*. Geneva: World Health Organisation.

Rifkin, S.B., Muller, F. and Bichmann, W. (1988) 'Primary health care: on measuring participation', *Social Science Medicine*, 26 (9): 931–40.

Riger, S. (1984) 'Vehicles for Empowerment: The case of Feminist Movement Organisations', in J. Rappaport (ed.), *Studies in Empowerment: steps toward understanding and action*. New York: Haworth Press: 99–117.

Rissel, C. (1994) 'Empowerment: the holy grail of health promotion?', *Health Promotion International*, 9 (1): 39–47.

Rissel, C.E., Perry, C.L., Wagenaar, A.C., Wolfson, M., Finnegan, J.R. and Komro, K.A. (1996a) 'Empowerment, alcohol, 8th grade students and health promotion', *Journal of Alcohol and Drug Education*, 41 (2): 105–19.

Rissel, C.E., Perry, C.L., and Finnegan, J.R. (1996b) 'Toward the assessment of psychological empowerment in health promotion: initial tests of validity and reliability', *Journal of the Royal Society of Health*, 116 (4): 211–18.

Ristock, J.L. and Pennell, J. (1996) *Community Research as Empowerment: Feminist links, postmodern interruptions*. New York: Oxford University Press.

Robertson, A. and Minkler, M. (1994) 'New health promotion movement: a critical examination', *Health Education Quarterly*, 21 (3): 295–312.

Robson, C. (1993) *Real World Research*. Oxford: Blackwell.

Rody, N. (1988) 'Empowerment as organisational policy in nutrition programs: A case study from the Pacific islands', *Journal of Nutrition Education*, 20 (3): 133–41.

Roethlisberger, F.J., Dickson, W.J. and Wright, H.A. (1947) *Management and the Worker*. Cambridge, MA: Harvard University Press.

Rootman, I. and Raeburn, J. (1994) 'The concept of health', in A. Pederson, M. O'Neill and I. Rootman (eds), *Health Promotion in Canada: Provincial, National and International Perspectives*. Toronto: W.B. Saunders. pp. 56–71.

Rose, S. (1986) 'Community Organisation: A survival strategy for community-based, empowerment-orientated programs', *Journal of Sociology and Social Welfare*, 13 (3): 491–506.

Roughan, J.J. (1986) *Village Organization for Development: Department of Political Science*. Honolulu: University of Hawaii. PhD.

Rudd, R.E. and Comings, J.P. (1994) 'Learner development materials: an empowerment product', *Health Education Quarterly*, 21 (3): 313–27.

Rudner-Lugo, N. (1996) 'Empowerment education: A case study of the resource sisters/companeras program', *Health Education Quarterly*, 23 (3): 281–9.

Sadan, E. and Churchman, A. (1996) 'Process-focused and product-focused community planning: Two variations of empowering professional practice', *Community Development Journal*, 32 (1): 3–16.

Salmen, L.F. (1994). 'The listening dimension of evaluation: Evaluation and Development'. Proceedings of the 1994 World Bank conference, World Bank Operations Evaluation Department.

Schmitt, D. and Weaver, D. (1979) *Leadership for Community Empowerment: A source book*. Midland, MI: Pendell.

Scrimgeour, D. (1997) *Community Control of Aboriginal Health Services in the Northern Territory*. Darwin: Menzies School of Health Research. Report 2, 1997.

Scriven, M. (1997) 'Book review. Empowerment Evaluation: Knowledge and tools for self-assessment and accountability', *Evaluation Practice*, 18 (2): 165–75.

Sechrest, L.E. (1997) 'Book review. Empowerment Evaluation: Knowledge and tools for self-assessment and accountability', *Environment and Behavior*, 29 (3): 422–26.

Seedhouse, D. (1997) *Health Promotion: Philosophy, Prejudice and Practice.* Chichester: John Wiley.

Seidman, S. and Wagner, D.G. (eds) (1992) *Postmodernism and Social Theory: The debate over general theory.* Oxford: Blackwell.

Seligman, M. (1975) *Helplessness: On Depression, Development and Death.* San Francisco, CA: W.H. Freeman.

Seligman, M. (1990) *Learned Optimism.* Toronto: Pocket Books.

Seligman, M. and Maier, S.F. (1967) 'Failure to escape traumatic shock', *Journal of Experimental Psychology,* 74: 1–9.

Serrano-Garcia, I. (1984) 'The Illusion of Empowerment: Community Development Within a Colonial Context', in J. Rappaport (ed.), *Studies in Empowerment: Steps toward understanding action.* New York: Haworth Press. pp. 173–200.

Shiva, V. (1991) *Ecology and the Politics of Survival: Conflicts over natural resources in India.* New Delhi: Sage.

Shrimpton, R. (1995) 'Community Participation in Food and Nutrition Programmes: An Analysis of Recent Governmental Experiences', in P. Pinstrup-Andersen, D. Pellitier and H. Alderman (eds), *Child Growth and Nutrition in Developing Countries: Priorities for action.* Ithaca, NY: Cornell University Press. pp. 243–61.

Simnett, I. (1995) *Managing Health Promotion: Developing healthy organisations and communities.* Chichester: John Wiley.

Simons-Morton, B.G. and Davis-Crump, A. (1996) 'Empowerment: the process and the outcome', *Health Education Quarterly,* 23 (3): 290–92.

Singh, R. (1994) 'Advocacy, empowerment and international collaboration. An experiment for rural development in India', *Indian Journal of Social Work,* 55 (3): 327–35.

Skocpol, T. (1993) 'The Potential Autonomy of the State', in M.E. Olsen and M.N. Marger (eds), *Power in Modern Societies.* San Francisco, CA: Westview Press. pp. 306–13.

Slocum, R., Wichhart, L., Rocheleau, D. and Thomas-Slayter, B. (1995) *Power, Process and Participation – Tools for Change.* London: Intermediate Technology Publications.

Smith, G.D. (1996) 'Income inequality and mortality: why are they related?', *British Medical Journal,* 312: 987–8.

Smith, G.D., Bartley, M. and Blane, D. (1990) 'The Black report on socioeconomic inequalities in health 10 years on', *British Medical Journal,* 301: 373–7.

Smithies, J. and Webster, G. (1998) *Community Involvement in Health.* Aldershot: Ashgate.

Snyder, M.M. and Doan, P.L. (1995) 'Who participates in the evaluation of international development aid?', *Evaluation Practice,* 16 (2): 141–52.

Speer, P. and Hughley, J. (1995) 'Community organising: An ecological route to empowerment and power', *American Journal of Community Psychology,* 23 (5): 729–48.

Speller, V., Learmonth, A. and Harrison, D. (1997) 'The search for evidence of effective health promotion', *British Medical Journal,* 315: 361–3.

Starfield, B. (2001) 'Improving equity in health: A research agenda' *International Journal of Health Services,* 31 (3): 545–66.

Starhawk, M.S. (1990) *Truth or Dare: Encounters with power, authority and mystery.* New York: HarperCollins.

Stevenson, H.M. and Burke, M. (1991) 'Bureaucratic logic in new social movement clothing: the limits of health promotion research', *Health Promotion International*, 6 (4): 281–90.

Stevenson, J.F., Mitchell, R.E. and Florin, P. (1996) 'Evaluation and self-direction in community-prevention coalitions', in D.M. Fetterman S.T. Kaftarian and A. Wandersman (eds), *Empowerment Evaluation: Knowledge and tools of self-assessment and accountability*. Thousand Oaks, CA: Sage. pp. 208–33.

Stewart, D.W. and Shamdasani, P.N. (1990) *Focus Groups: Theory and practice*. London: Sage.

Strawn, C. (1994) 'Beyond the buzz word: empowerment in community outreach and education', *Journal of Applied Behavioural Science*, 30 (2): 159–74.

Streefland, P.H. (1996) 'Mutual support arrangements among the poor in South Asia', *Community Development Journal*, 31 (4): 302–28.

Strong, G. (1998) 'The gentle art of defeating a giant', *The Age*, 21 November: 10.

Stufflebeam, D. (1994) 'Empowerment evaluation, objectivist evaluation and evaluation standards: where the future of evaluation should not go and where it needs to go', *Evaluation Practice*, 15 (3): 321–38.

Sutherland, R. (2002) 'Community development and health work in Northern Ireland: Context, history and development', in L. Adams, M. Amos and J. Munro (eds), *Promoting Health: Politics and practice*. London: Sage.

Swift, C. and Levin, G. (1987) 'Empowerment: an emerging mental health technology', *Journal of Primary Prevention*, 8 (1 and 2): 71–94.

Syme, L. (1997) 'Individual vs Community Interventions in Public Health Practice: Some Thoughts about a New Approach', *Vichealth Letter*, July (2): 2–9.

Tannahill, A. (1985) 'What is health promotion?', *Health Education Journal*, 44 (4): 167–8.

Taylor, R. and Rieger, A. (1985) 'Medicine as a social science: Rudolf Virchow on the typhus epidemic in Upper Silesia', *International Journal of Health Services*, 15: 547–59.

Taylor, V. (1995) 'Social Reconstruction and Community Development in the Transition to Democracy in South Africa', in G. Craig and M. Mayo (eds), *Community Empowerment: A reader in participation and development*. London: Zed Books. pp. 168–80.

Tones, K., Tilford, S. and Keeley Robinson, Y. (1990) *Health Education: Effectiveness and Efficiency*. London: Chapman and Hall.

Tonon, M.A. (1980) 'Concepts in community empowerment: a case of sanitary change in a Guatemalan village', *International Journal of Health Education*, 23 (4): 1–16.

Toronto Department of Public Health (1991a) *Health Inequalities in the City of Toronto*. Toronto: Department of Public Health.

Toronto Department of Public Health (1991b) *Advocacy for Basic Health Prerequisites: Policy Report*. Toronto: Department of Public Health.

Torre, D. (1986) 'Empowerment: Structured conceptualisation and instrument development'. PhD, Cornell University.

Townsend, P. (1986) 'Why are the many poor?', *International Journal of Health Services*, 16 (1): 1–32.

Trice Gray, S. (1998) *Evaluation with Power: A new approach to organizational effectiveness, empowerment and excellence*. San Francisco, CA: Jossey-Bass.

Tudor-Smith, C. and Farley, P. (1997) 'The future of health promotion', in L. Jones and M. Sidell (eds), *The challenge of promoting health: Exploration and action*. London: MacMillan. pp. 278–80.

Turbyne, J. (1996) 'The Enigma of Empowerment: A Study of the Transformation of Concepts in Policy Making Processes'. PhD, University of Bath.

Uphoff, N. (1990) 'Paraprojects as New Modes of International Development Assistance', *World Development* 18 (10): 1401–11.

Uphoff, N. (1991) 'A field methodology for participatory self-education', *Community Development Journal*, 26 (4): 271–85.

Valadez, J. and Bamberger, M. (1994) *Monitoring and Evaluating Social Programs in Developing Countries: A handbook for policymakers, managers and researchers*. Washington DC: World Bank Publications.

Valvarde, C. (1991) *Critical Theory in health education*. Montreal: Montreal DSC.

Vargas, L.V. (1991) 'Reflections on methodology of evaluation', *Community Development Journal*, 26 (4): 266–70.

Vasoo, S. (1991) 'Grass-root Mobilisation and Citizen Participation: Issues and Challenges', *Community Development Journal*, 26 (1): 1–7.

Vindhya, U. and Kalpana, V. (1988) 'Voluntary organisations and women's struggle for change: experience with BCT', *Indian Journal of Social Work*, 50 (2): 183–97.

Wadsworth, Y. and McGuiness, M. (1992) *Understanding Anytime: A consumer evaluation of acute psychiatric hospitals*. Melbourne VMIAC.

Wallerstein, N. (1992) 'Powerlessness, empowerment and health: Implications for health promotion programs', *American Journal of Health Promotion*, 6 (3): 197–205.

Wallerstein, N. and Bernstein, E. (1988) 'Empowerment education: Freire's ideas adapted to health education', *Health Education Quarterly*, 15 (4): 379–94.

Wallerstein, N. and Bernstein, E. (1994) 'Introduction to community empowerment: Participatory education and health', *Health Education Quarterly*, 21 (2): 171–86.

Wallerstein, N. and Sanchez-Merki, V. (1994) 'Freirian praxis in health education: research results from an adolescent prevention program', *Health Education: Theory and practice*, 9 (1): 105–18.

Wang, C. and Burris, M. (1994) 'Empowerment through photo novella: Portraits of participants', *Health Education Quarterly*, 21 (2): 171–86.

Ward, J. (1987) 'Community development with marginal people: the role of conflict', *Community Development Journal*, 22 (1): 18–21.

Wartenberg, T.E. (1990) *The Forms of Power: From domination to transformation*. Philadelphia, PA: Temple University Press.

Weber, M. (1947) *The Theory of Social and Economic Organization*. New York: The Free Press.

Wegelin-Schuringa, M. (1992) *Participation Approaches to Urban Water Supply and Sanitation*. The Hague: IRC.

Werner, D. (1988) 'Empowerment and health', *Contact. Christian Medical Commission*, 102: 1–9.

Wheat, S. (1997) (April) Banking on a better future, *Guardian Weekly*. 9th February: 19.

Whitehead, M. (1991) 'The concepts and principles of equity and health', *Health Promotion International*, 6 (3): 217–28.

Wilkinson, R. (1986) 'Income and Mortality', in R. Wilkinson (ed.) *Class and Health: Research and Longitudinal Data*. London: Tavistock.

Wilkinson, R. (1996) *Unhealthy Societies: The Afflictions of Inequality*. New York: Routledge.

World Health Organisation (1978) *Declaration of Alma Ata*. Geneva: World Health Organisation.

World Health Organisation (1986) *Ottawa Charter for Health Promotion*. Geneva: World Health Organisation.

World Health Organisation (2002a) 'Conference statement. The Adelaide Recommendations' available at www.who.int/hpr (accessed 6 June 2002).

World Health Organisation (2002b) 'Sundsvall Statement On Supportive Environments For Health' available at www.who.int/hpr (accessed 6 June 2002).

World Health Organisation (2002c) 'The Jakarta Declaration on Leading Health Promotion into the 21st Century' available at www.who.int/hpr (accessed 6 June 2002).

World Health Organisation (2002d) 'Mexico Global Conference for Health Promotion' available at www.who.int/hpr (accessed 6 June 2002).

Wrong, D.H. (1988) *Power: Its forms, bases and uses*. Chicago, IL: The University of Chicago Press.

Yeo, M. (1993) 'Toward an ethic of empowerment for health promotion', *Health Promotion International*, 8 (3): 225–35.

Youker, R. and Burnett, N.R. (1993) 'The Project Cycle and the Project Appraisal Process', in ESCAP (eds), *Selected readings on project planning*. New York: United Nations. pp. 51–58.

Zakus, J.D.L. and Lysack, C.L. (1998) 'Revisiting community participation', *Health Policy and Planning*, 13 (1): 1–12.

Zimmerman, M.A. and Rappaport, J. (1988) 'Citizen participation, perceived control and psychological empowerment', *American Journal of Community Psychology*, 16 (5): 725–43.

Zimmerman, M.A. and Zahniser, J.H. (1991) 'Refinements of sphere-specific measures of perceived control: development of a socio-political control scale', *Journal of Community Psychology*, 19 (April): 189–204.

Index